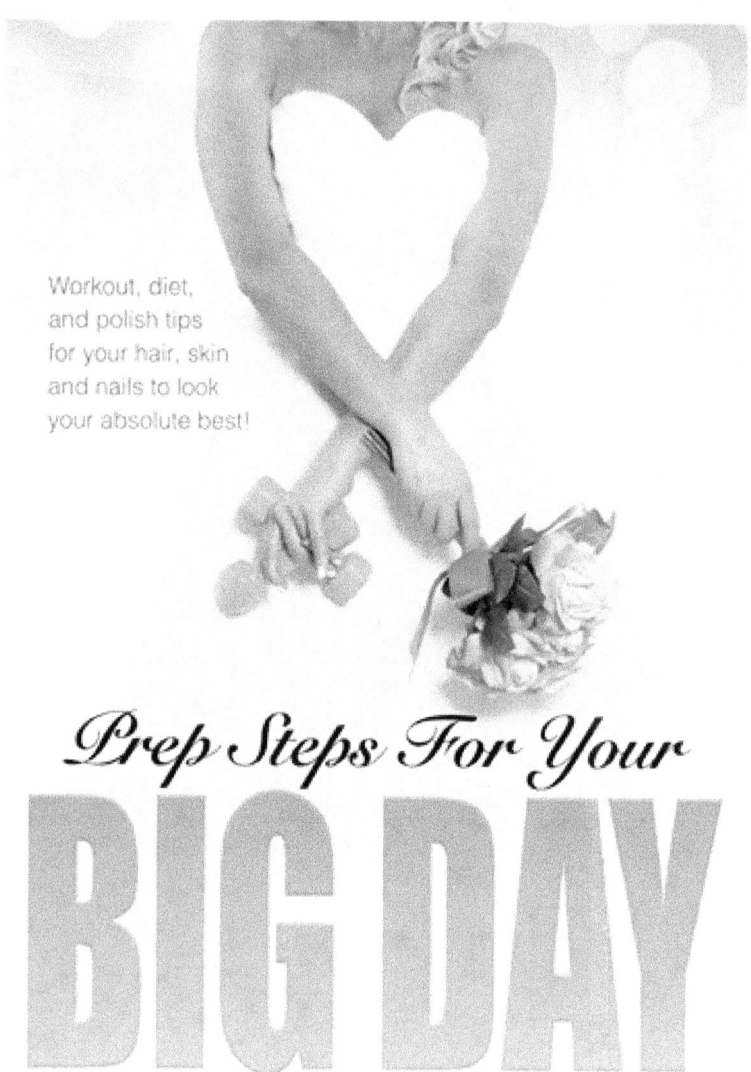

Workout, diet, and polish tips for your hair, skin and nails to look your absolute best!

Prep Steps For Your

BIG DAY

Table of Contents

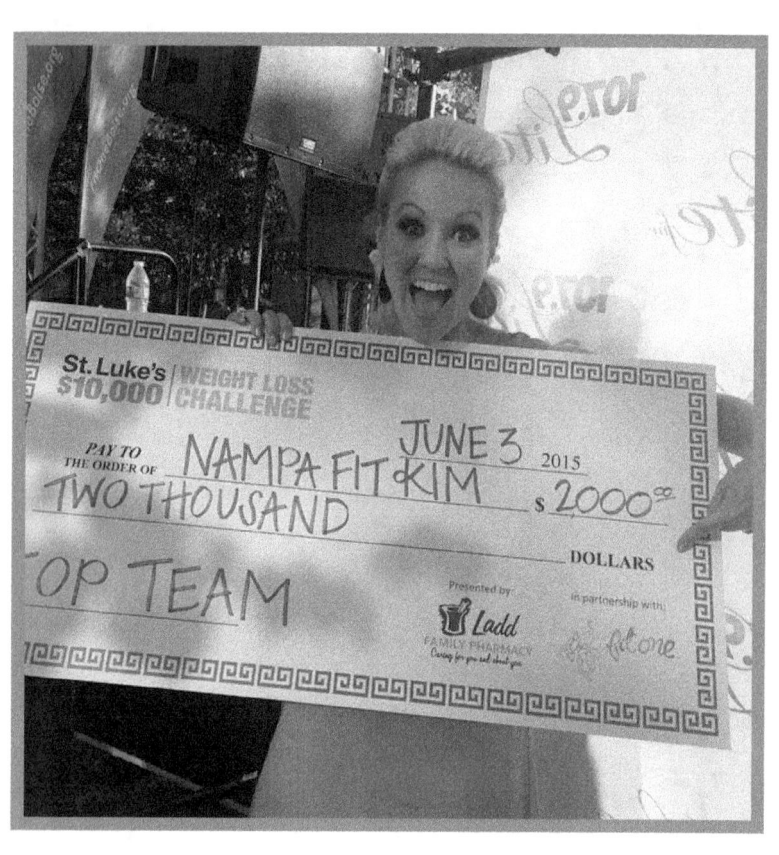

Nice to Meet You!

I didn't grow up as an athlete. Like, at all. I've never played sports, never won anything, and never really saw the need for fitness until later in life. What discovering my passion later taught me is that it's never *too* late to have a healthier life.

Since then, I've held just about every job one can in the fitness industry, from mopping the gym floors to teaching group fitness, personal training to owning a studio, and most recently, Director of a 20,000-member facility. I studied Communications at Boise State University; I am a Master Trainer for the National Academy of Sports Medicine and have coached the 1st place team five years in a row in the $10,000 Canyon County Weight Loss Challenge. With the program's success in Idaho, I was honored to launch the challenge in Kitsap County, Washington when we moved back to my hometown in 2016.

I've been a personal trainer for over 15 years and worked as Master Trainer for the National Academy of Sports Medicine to get new personal trainers started in their careers. Some people get into fitness for the free gym membership or with hopes of being the next Miss Olympia, but to me, personal training is about so much more than the latest workout craze. Trust me, when you own a gym everyone wants to sell you the latest craze. In my tenure, I've studied behavioral change, nutrition, and eating disorders including food addiction and the extreme opposite. I've worked with clients and their doctors for help with neuromuscular disorders and taught classes for folks with

Special Needs. And my most passionate work was when I was working with obese and morbidly obese individuals.

Along with all of that, in my career, I've helped hundreds of clients prepare for various Big Days: a wife preparing for her husband's return from deployment, dozens of stressed out brides-to-be. I've even helped a gentlemen prepare to meet his online crush face-to-face after a year-long courtship and a Mrs. America contestant. I myself was a top ranking fitness competitor and I've helped several others take the stage since. So you see, your Big Day can be just about any event that's important to you and that you want to look great for.

Losing some weight or getting the workout figured out is just one part, but true confidence comes when you know you're going to shine on your Big Day– so we'll work to get your skin, hair and bod all looking amazing, so when your Big Day comes, you will be your most radiant self!

How to Use This Book for Your Big Day

This book is broken down by weeks out from the Big Day. Each week will be broken down into the 3 main things you'll need to focus on: your workout, your diet, and (my favorite) your polish – all of the finishing touches for your hair, skin and nails to make you look flawless for your Big Day. We're not talking about slapping on some lip-gloss and calling it good – I'm going to show you how to actually make your hair and skin healthier so that your make-up goes on smoother, your tan lasts longer, and your overall presents is... well... polished.

The first chapter will discuss what you should be focusing on if you are 10 weeks out from GO TIME. Chapter two will cover your 9 weeks out focus and so on and so on. But remember, each chapter will build upon the last. You will completely master the tools in the first week and they will stick with you as you change your focus for the next week. Some of the diet or habit changes will be easy to plug into your life but others might take more than a week to fully integrate, and that's okay! If the skills in one particular section aren't quite sticking (or maybe you're a crazed bridezilla with a million other things pulling your attention) you can take another week or so to focus on it. But do continue to move on to the next section to keep on track with the timeline until your Big Day.

Now, if you picked up this book in a pinch and only have a few weeks to get ready, don't worry. You can jump in at the chapter that is within the right time frame for you, but I recommend going back and reading the entire book. It may be a bit harder to make big changes in less time, but you'll be amazed at how strong your will to change is when you realize that your butt is going to be in a bikini or wedding dress in just a few weeks!

Of course I am a personal trainer and fitness expert and I do believe in creating healthy habits to last a lifetime. In fact, I have helped hundreds of clients make life-long changes. I'm not one for quick fixes, magic pills or potions, yo-yo dieting or anything dangerous. There are hundreds of books and resources out there with incredible tips to help make life-long changes, but this book isn't one of them. This book is to get you looking great for your time in the spot-light, whatever that may be. One of the fortunate side effects is that you'll be so impressed with the results that you will keep some of these changes in your daily life- and even if you do let some slide for a while, you'll be educated enough to do it again when the need arises and if you forget – just flip to the 'Weeks Out' chapter you need and get started again. Or better yet, after you've followed the plan and breezed through your Big Day looking polished and fabulous, start planning another one so you stay motivated to keep looking fantastic!

And if you don't have a Big Day in the works – make one! Book the photographer! Buy the tickets! Reserve the room! Shop for the outfit! Sign up for the race! When an end date is real and in sight, it becomes your motivation when the morning alarm goes off. It becomes easier to pass on the fries and get inspired for the workout. So here we go, it's time to start prepping for your Big Day!

10

10 WEEKS OUT

10 WEEKS WORKOUT

Choose Your Weapons!

Did you really think you were going to get a lean, toned, and beautiful body without adding exercise to the mix? Sorry.

You are about to read something that may break your heart. It may force you to rethink everything you have ever believed. Brace yourself - Here it goes: There is no magic pill, potion, drop, bar, vitamin, shake, mix, rub, lotion, wrap, shoes, pants, or bra that is going to give you the body you want. I know, bummer right? It's time to take off your blinders and really think about the advertising messages you have been force-fed your entire life. You have been lied to. A lot.

Remember the butt-shaping shoe epidemic? These hideous contraptions were not only old-lady ugly but in fact hazardous to your ankles, knees, and arches. The "good ones" cost over one-hundred dollars and had a rounded bottom, creating instability, which, in theory, was supposed to make your buns work harder while walking. Usually the women who have fallen victim to this footwear fraud would have benefited from just a walk in general, no ugly shoes needed.

As a trainer, I can't think of a single beneficial exercise where rocking your feet would help anything. In fact, when I do have clients show up to trainings or classes wearing those butt-shaping shams they are asked to change because 1) they

Prep Steps for Your Big Day

increase your risk for injury by having such an unstable base and 2) they are so ugly, I fear it may distract others...Just kidding.

By the way, since their inception, Reebok, New Balance and countless other shoe makers have been forced to pay out millions of dollars in settlements ranging from false advertising to medical bills for wearers who sustained injury.

The point is, there truly is no quick-fix. You have to do some work. But don't worry – it doesn't have to suck and when your Big Day rolls around you'll be so glad you did. We are, quite literally, building your body so this is the week that you choose your weapons of mass construction!

Maybe you join a gym. Maybe you start going to that gym you've been paying for the last 8 months. Maybe you find a steal on craigslist for some weights for your garage. It doesn't matter where you do it, but it does matter how you do it and how often.

You'll have two options throughout this book. The first is the Print & Go Workouts – these are for anyone heading to the gym with workouts using machines found in most fitness facilities. The second option is the Print & Stay Workouts. These are for the people who have some supplies at home, like free weights. If you don't have access to either, you're going to have to make some sort of investment. The bottom line is, to get the body you want YOU HAVE TO LIFT WEIGHTS.

This week, your focus is to learn your body and where your fitness and strength levels are It's the same thing you would do if you hired a trainer, heck it's the same thing I would do if you came to me!

You will have a list of exercises and a range for a starting weight. If you're a new girl, start with that recommended weight, if you've already been at this a while, try the Fit Chick weights or higher. Keep in mind you need to be able to complete the move 12 times. No I didn't just make that **num**ber up, it has significance that you'll learn about later.

I think the two of the scariest things about walking into a gym or investing in a home weight set are:

1) not knowing what to do

2) not knowing which weight to start with

This week, you'll learn how to battle those two scary things. Say you've seen a great arm-toning video on Instagram and you want to try it out, but the meat-head in the photo is lifting a Volkswagen in each arm. So here do YOU start? I've helped so many people who are just starting out that I can almost always pinpoint their strength level. It's like my own super-power.

The great thing is, you don't have to guess – you have try. Don't sell yourself short. Remember, you have probably lifted a gallon of milk (2lbs). If you're a mommy, I know you can fling around a car-seat like it's a feather (20lbs). And if you've ever carried a load of groceries in one trip, you are stronger than you think.

On our first day of training, I ask my clients "If you had to choose a weight to do (insert any exercise) with, which weight would you choose?" Of course I remind them that they have to perform the exercise 12 times.

 Most of the time women have no idea how much weight they are capable of lifting. If they do make a choice they almost always choose to light of weight and instead of 12, they end up doing the exercise hundreds of times before they realize that they probably could have gone with heavier weight. So barring any injuries, these starting weights will work. Use this guide at the gym this week to help you choose which weights you're going to use moving forward or, as I call it, choose your weapons! Column one is the exercise, if you're not sure what it is – turn to my site www.kimatthegym.com.

Column two is the weight range, New Girl is the lightest.

DO NOT go any lighter that this weight (even if you think I'm crazy)! Most bags of cat/dog food weight more than you think, you can lift this weight.

If you're already active and know your way around the weight room use the Fit Chick weight as your starting point.

In the third column write in which weight you actually used. This step is so vital because we are going to need this information for your workouts in the coming weeks.

A great way to tackle this week is to do your lower body exercises one day and all of your upper body exercises the next day. On days three and four, just repeat what you've already done - just to be sure you've chosen the right weights!

Don't forget - You have to be able to lift that weight 12 times. Let me be clear ONLY 12 times.

1) If you can lift it more than 15 times, your weight is to light. Go heavier.

2) If you can't do the exercise at least 8 times, quit showing off. Your weight is too heavy. Go lighter.

The goal is to be getting in tune with your body. You cannot move forward if you don't even know where you're starting. So don't be scared – just walk right up to that weight rack or the weight section of your sporting goods store and choose your weapons!

PRINT & GO

Exercise	Recommended Start Range New Girl—Fit Chick	Try it! Then Fill in the Weight You Can Lift 12 Times
Example: Bicep curl	8 lbs—15 lbs	10 lbs
Overhead Triceps Extension	5 lbs—12 lbs	
Shoulder Press	5 lbs—15 lbs	
Chest Press	8 lbs—20 lbs	
Leg Extension	30 lbs—50lbs	
Hamstring Curl	10 lbs—30 lbs	

WORKOUT

Exercise	Recommended Start Range New Girl—Fit Chick	Try it! Then Fill in the Weight You Can Lift 12 Times
Chest Fly Machine	20 lbs—50 lbs	
Seated Row	15 lbs—45 lbs	
Bent Row	15 lbs—30 lbs	
Frontal Shoulder Raise	3 lbs—8 lbs	
Lat Pull-Down	20 lbs—50lbs	
Seated Leg Press	30 lbs—90 lbs	

PRINT & STAY

Exercise	Recommended Start Range New Girl—Fit Chick	Try it! Then Fill in the Weight You Can Lift 12 Times
Example: Bicep curl	8 lbs—15 lbs	10 lbs
Overhead Triceps Extension	5lbs—12 lbs	
Shoulder Press	5 lbs—15 lbs	
Chest Press	8 lbs—20 lbs	
Squat	10 lbs—50lbs	
Straight Leg Deadl-Lift	10 lbs—30 lbs	

WORKOUT

Exercise	Recommended Start Range New Girl—Fit Chick	Try it! Then Fill in the Weight You Can Lift 12 Times
Chest Fly	8 lbs—50 lbs	10 lbs
Upright Row	5 lbs—45 lbs	
Bent Row	15 lbs—35 lbs	
Frontal Shoulder Raise	3 lbs—8 lbs	
Push-Ups (On your toes!)	10 lbs—50lbs	
Hands Close Push-Ups	How Many Can You Do?	
Plank (Knees or toes)	How Long Can You Hold? (secs)	

10 WEEKS OUT DIET

Don't Get Wrapped Up

I have heard some of the silliest "health tips" from clients. People pick up the strangest things from their body-builder cousins or their 90-pound co-worker or from whatever diet craze is hot right now. Usually there is one small glimmer of truth in the fad but it gets stretched out to the extreme. For example, Cayenne pepper really is a thermogenic, meaning it increases your calorie burning ability on a microscopic, teeny-tiny level...but a 3-day cayenne-only cleanse? Noooooo! Please don't fall victim to these crazy extremes add a little cayenne to some favorite recipes you'll get the same benefits without doing anything crazy.

For the next 10 weeks I am going to ask you to simply tune it all out. Go back to the basics with me for a while and don't get wrapped up in the details of the food labels, or glycemic index, or counting calories or carbs, or tricks from your bodybuilder cousin. Stay focused on your big picture, your Big Day and as we progress we'll get into the smaller details to get you into that smaller dress. Hopefully by the end of this journey you'll have a much clearer picture to be able to differentiate facts from nonsense.

I know a lot of people would expect the diet to get really intense, really quickly - since 10 weeks isn't that much time and the biggest day of your life it just around the corner. So here you go: You've got 10 weeks...promise to eat only veggies and don't look at any French fries until after the Big Day and you're all set!

Good luck with that.

In my experience (with all different kinds of clients), it just doesn't work. People jump in and go full-throttle with a new "diet" and force themselves to eat celery and rice cakes for a week, maybe even two but by week 3 they've given into life's little cravings, (totally normal by the way) but instead of making any progress to get into the bathing suit, they feel like a failure and shift their focus onto what color wrap their going to buy to go over the bathing suit.

So don't go cleaning out your cupboards just yet, after all we still have 10 weeks and if you master to this week's diet focus before you move on to the next, you'll be building great habits and lean muscle while losing excess fat. Remember each week of your diet and workouts will build upon the week before so by the time your Big Day arrives, you'll love what you see in the mirror!

So for now just focus on what needs to get done THIS WEEK and don't get wrapped up in the details!

I'm sure you've heard the saying that "breakfast is the most important meal of the day. Well, not this week. This week, your only focus is on your pre and post workout meals. Choosing the right fuel in before your workouts and repairing your body after your workouts, are truly the most important decisions you can make this week.
You may be feeling like the week 10 workout wasn't all that hard, after all you only had to do 12 of everything – but if you did do the work and took the time to find the right weights, then it still qualifies as a work out! So honor your body by preparing it correctly and replenishing it right.

THE FIRST MOST IMPORTANT MEAL OF THE DAY: PRE-WORKOUT

What is the first thing you think of when you see the word carb?

Bread?

Pasta?

Rolls?

But do you know what else a carbohydrate is? Fruits and veggies! Contrary to popular belief a carb (or carbohydrate) is not the devil. It's true, the grain that is used to make the bread is a carbohydrate and it's really good for your body. Sadly all of the crap that food manufacturers add to that grain to turn it into bread deafens it's positive effects and brings in a whole bunch of negative ones and you'll learn more on choosing good breads/pastas shortly. So when you see that skinny-minny co-worker who swears she lost all her weight by avoiding carbs, she's lying. What she means to say is that she avoided BREAD products, not carbs.

So from now on when you see the word carb or carbohydrate in this book, I am referring to fruits, veggies and whole grains – NOT just bread and pasta.

There are lots of 'low-carb' plans out there and they may help you lose some weight if you're not interested in exercising-but you! You have a Big Day to prepare for and as you've already learned, not exercising is not an option. You will exercise and you will need those carbs.

Now, what does a carb really do for you? Think of them as the match that starts the fat-burning fire. They give you the boost of energy you need to get you ready to head to the gym. Much like putting gas in your gas tank, you'll be able to go just a few miles further if you top it off before you hit the road. So about an hour before you head to the gym focus on getting a great source of carbs to get you fired up and ready to work!

A HEALTHY PRE-WORKOUT MEAL IS...

Any and all fruits

Yes, there are some that rank a little higher on the glycemic index, which means they have a higher sugar content but don't get all wrapped up in that. Just get fruit in your body. If you don't like bananas, here's a simple tip: don't eat bananas! Go for whatever you like. You can slice it, dice it, juice it, leave the skin on, peel the skin off whatever it takes to get it in your body. No, you may not dip it in chocolate or sugar.

A HEALTHY PRE-WORKOUT MEAL IS...

Any and all veggies

Yes, there is a difference between fibrous carbohydrates and starchy carbohydrates but don't get all wrapped up in that. If you don't like broccoli, here's another simple tip: don't eat broccoli! Go for whatever you like and again – you can juice them, steam them, eat them whole, chop them up- whatever is going to get it into your body. Just don't dip them in ranch dressing or deep-fat-fry them.

A HEALTHY PRE-WORKOUT MEAL IS...

Whole grains.

Spending a few hours in the bread isle is always a fun way to spend an afternoon! Just kidding. It's like one of those terrible nightmares where you're stuck in a giant spider web, except all around you are stickers and labels strewn with the words "Nutritious Whole Grains" and "Healthy" and "Hearty." But next time you're in the store, flip over one of those pretty little liars and look at the first word in the ingredient list.

31

Chances are you'll have to flip a bunch of them over…because most of them are LYING! If the first word in the ingredient list is not the word "Whole" put it down. It means that the whole grain has been tampered with, bleached, enriched or otherwise doesn't exist in the food that is in that package. The drag is, even if the grain has been tampered with, food labels can still brag about having 'nutritious whole grains' because at one point it did or maybe it still does somewhere buried deep in the ingredients. Unfortunately, all that other stuff does not serve well for your pre-workout fuel.

This first word check works for everything – when you're shopping for pastas, bagels, crackers, oatmeal, cereals etc. After making sure the first word is "whole," move down that food label, and check the sugar content. If it has more than 8 grams of sugar put it down and go find something else.

Don't get wrapped up with the gimmicks on the front of the package and don't get wrapped up in calories – you're on your way to gym to burn them off anyways. The good stuff is out there though, just take the time to look and when you get to know which cereals, pastas, and snacks are the good ones you'll do better at stocking your cupboards with great pre-workout fuel.

A HEALTHY PRE-WORKOUT MEAL IS...

About the size of your hands

Easy enough right? An apple fits in your hands, maybe two if they're small. A banana could be broken into both hands. A slice of whole grain toast is about the size of your hand. Two big handfuls of veggies would be a good sized salad. Keep it simple. Don't get wrapped up in measuring or weighing things. You don't even have to dirty a dish! Just get all of this awesome jet fuel in your body and get going!

A HEALTHY PRE-WORKOUT MEAL IS NOT...

Fried, dairy, sloshy, salty, buttery, fatty, sugary or any- thing that makes you feel heavy, full and lazy.

.

THE SECOND MOST IMPORTANT MEAL OF THE DAY: POST-WORKOUT REPLENISH

During your first week of exercise you haven't had to do much heavy lifting. That was on purpose. We need to get you in the habit of working out 3-4 times a week, a daunting task if you're not already a gym goer. But with the motivation of your Big Day lurking in the background of your mind, hopefully you're finding the inspiration you need to get you there.

Maybe you didn't get to the gym as often as you'd like, that's okay. Even if your workout was just a walk through the dog park, treat it like gym time and eat the right fuel before and give yourself the right reward after. If you can do that 3-4 times a week, that's still 6-8 meals a week that we know are on the right track!

So, you got some sort of workout in. You're awesome! You're sweaty. You're energized. You're...starving! You want to treat yourself to something for all that hard work so you hop into your favorite coffee shop for a tasty, frozen something and maybe a blueberry muffin (because that seems healthier than a cake-pop). WRONG! Do NOT reward yourself with treats. YOU ARE NOT A DOG. Within just a few sips you'll have undone all of that beautiful work and you will erase the entire workout. Continue eating and drinking that sugary, lard-laden garbage and you'll have set yourself back a day or two.

So what do you eat? The most important thing to remember is that the window of time following your workout is one of the most opportune times to feed your body the things it loves the most: nutrients and protein! After all of that energy expenditure on your walk, swim, in the gym, or in your favorite fitness class, your body is doing amazing metabolic things, even long after you've left the gym. The best thing you can do to reward yourself is feed it something that will repair the damaged tissue. This is not done with a dainty little iceberg lettuce salad one might think is a healthy choice after a workout, it is done with protein.

With every weight you lift or step you take, there are hundreds of tiny muscle explosions that create heat and that's when you get sweaty! It takes stored calories (a.k.a. fat) to create that heat, hence the phrase "burning fat". Along with that heat comes damage to the tissue. That shredded up tissue is part of what makes you sore the next day and a big reason why most people quit a fitness routine before they see any results. It hurts! But only because they don't know how to repair that damaged tissues. Sometimes my clients (and also my husband) think that whining about how sore you are will fix it…I'd have to double check, but I'm pretty sure it doesn't.

After your workout, picture each gram of protein you eat entering your body like little construction workers. They will go to the site of the damage and rebuild that tissue back stronger, and more dense then it was before – thus the creation of lean mass. You won't feel as sore and you'll have rewarded yourself with something that actually serves your body and moves you toward your goals instead of further away from them.

One of the last things I ask of (or yell at) my clients on their way out the door is: "DO NOT WASTE THIS WORKOUT!" One of the worst things you can do is go home and eat something fatty or sugary. Or even more damaging- eat nothing at all- because then, all of the amazing changes you just made won't stay (they never got repaired by the construction workers remember?) So be mindful when choosing your post-workout meals, that you are rewarding yourself with nutrients to help keep the changes, not undo them.

Prep Steps for Your Big Day

A HEALTHY POST WORKOUT MEAL IS:

A great source of lean protein

Chicken breast, fish, eggs/egg whites, turkey, pork tenderloin, elk, bison. Remember, each little amino-acid molecule found in these types of food rush to the muscle and repair any damage. Eating this will reduce your soreness and allow your muscle to heal quickly and stronger than before. Since you won't be as sore you'll be more likely to get back to your workout the next day.

A HEALHTY POST WORKOUT MEAL IS...

A good protein shake or meal replacement bar

Here is a warning about these items. YOU CAN NOT LIVE ON THEM. Refer back to the beginning of the chapter. There is no magic shake or bar! But they do serve their purpose when you're in a pinch post-workout. It's tough to rush home and grill up a steak after each workout so I do encourage you to find easy ways to supplement for your busy life.

Always try to choose whole foods first and if you must reach for a shake or bar limit it to only this time of day (post workout). Also, be sure to watch out for sugars and fat content of those quick fixes, most are loaded with sugar or artificial sweeteners. Look for no more than 8 grams of sugar. With total fat, no more than 3 grams. I'm going to repeat that to make it very clear: no more than 8 grams of sugar and no more than 3 grams of total fat.

Don't get wrapped up in saturated fat vs unsaturated, trans fat, mono, poly… just look at the line that says TOTAL FAT – if it is more than 3 grams, try to look for a better brand.

I'm not very brand loyal, I buy whatever is on sale (as long as the fat and sugar is low), but I ALWAYS have one handy.

There is a ton to choose from so if your face is contorting as you recall the "muscle drinks" of the 80's, maybe it's time to visit your neighborhood nutrition store again. Don't get wrapped up in the marketing of what brand is the best – it all serves the same purpose and there are a million different flavors and options. Some offer protein from soy, whey, rice, even hemp. So do a little shopping, try a few flavors and brands until you find one that meets your needs and your taste buds.

A HEALTHY POST WORKOUT MEAL IS...

Loaded with nutrients

Post-workout is the time to give your body all of the things it needs. Load up super-foods like green, leafy veggies and colorful fruit but don't forget the protein! Along with this serving of fruits and veggies grab something that will repair the muscle to; things like hummus, Greek yogurt, almonds all carry power-packed protein and go great with fruits and veggies.

A HEALTHY POST WORKOUT MEAL IS **NOT**...

Fried, doughy, sugary, salty, dairy, fatty, or anything that does not offer protein or nutrients, i.e., a salad of iceberg lettuce.

You have one week to master these two meals. If you're already a regular exerciser, this shouldn't be that hard to incorporate. If you're new to the exercise scene, remember that at this point EVERYTHING counts as exercise: a 15-minute walk, a home fitness DVD, a bike ride, a play-date kicking a soccer ball at the park, a gym session, a golf game – all of it. So treat it as such and honor your body with the proper pre/post workout meals. You'll quickly notice that your time spent wasn't so bad, you won't be as sore so you'll be more likely to stick with it, and your meal planning will start to come together. After this week's focus you'll have much better footing as you move into the following weeks. So remember, we've got 10 weeks until your Big Day so for right now,

Do not waste your workout!
Do not get wrapped up in the details!

10 WEEKS OUT POLISH

Beating the Free Radical Bully
and the Nectar of the Gods

L et's say your Big Day is your husband coming home after months on military deployment. He hasn't touched a woman's skin in God-knows-how-long and all he can think about is getting his hands on you! He can't wait to see your beautiful skin and kiss every inch of your body.

Are you going to take a shower, shave, and call it good?

I don't know what your Big Day is but I can tell you that razor burn is NEVER sexy. Nor is a hairy upper lip, or worse, breaking out on your upper lip from a waxing experiment gone amiss.

We start RIGHT NOW, 10 weeks out, with some simple prep work to get your hair, skin and nails looking healthy, strong, and beautiful from the inside out.

   1.) Water. Water. Water. Or, as I like to call it, The Nectar of the Gods!

   Dehydration is one of the biggest culprits behind dark eye circles, dull skin, and blotchiness. It's not even so much the dehydration as much as it is the alcohol (both the kind we slather on our face in cleansers or the kind we shoot at the bar), the sun, and the poor food choices we make.

Prep Steps for Your Big Day

Even aspirin and spicy foods can expand your blood vessels making your skin look red and splotchy. So increasing your water intake will help schlep off some of that stuff from the inside out and be a great first step in preparing your skin for your Big Day. The bad news is you can't chug a gallon the night before your Big Day and wake up blemish free. You have to start NOW!

A great rule of thumb is to drink as many ounces of water per day as what your ideal body weight is in pounds. So let's say your currently 150lbs, but by your Big Day you would like to be 130lbs, you should aim to consume at least 130 ounces of water per day. That's a lot, a full gallon of water a day. But it can be done and if you want to look your best it must be done!

A few tips make sure water is a critical part of your beauty regimen:

- Fill a glass and set it by your bedside at night – the moment the alarm goes off, chug that sucker! I always feel like if miss the mark on my water intake for the entire rest of the day; at least I know I got SOMETHING in first thing. You could even add a little slice of lemon for an added antioxidant bonus (more on that to come)

- Buy a gallon jug of water and make tic marks or a timeline on it with a permanent marker to let you know when it's time to drink. For example by 3:00pm, you should be half-way through the gallon if you have any hope of finishing it before bed time. You could also write motivational words like "Almost There" or "Keep Drinking – You're getting married in 10 weeks!" You could even bedazzle that bugger if you wanted so it looks pretty sitting on your desk – it's going to be there a while!

If you can't stand room temperature H2O, fill your jug with a cup or two of water and then freeze it overnight. The ice on the bottom will keep your youth serum cool all day.

- If you can't stand the taste, drop in a few thinly sliced cumbers, lemons, or berries.

2.) The other big (and very important) focus for this week is introducing a good antioxidant vitamin into your Big Day budget. Beauty companies make billions of dollars selling creams, potions, lotions and makeup designed to cover up and fix your blemishes. But what we're going to do is clear your skin, even out your tone, reduce redness/blotchiness, and give you a gorgeous glow from the inside out! But that doesn't happen overnight. It may take a few days or maybe even a few weeks before you really see the results on the outside but believe me, amazing things will be happening on the inside.

I'm sure you've heard that a diet rich in antioxidants is great for your health. It reduces your risk of cancer, keeps your immune system strong, and yes, may assist in your weight loss efforts. So why then am I putting this vital tip in the 'polish' section? Because the science of what is happening on a molecular level is amazing and will give your skin the strength and re-salience it needs to stay looking healthy and beautiful, especially if you plan to get a pretty glow the old-fish-ironed way – sun tanning. We'll talk about more about ways to get a natural looking tan as we get closer to the Big Day.

An antioxidant is any chemical that can neutralize a free radical. So picture the school bully, he's a lone wolf. A free radical is a bad cell chemical that got loose in your body from eating some not-so-nutritious processed foods or staying out in the sun to long, or maybe you just happen to live on planet earth where toxins are always bombarding you.

So this free radical bully is hanging out in your body causing a ruckus everywhere he goes, creating wrenkales, sagging, and UV damage. He also slows your body's recovery time so that little tiny pimple that used to clear up over-night now seems to hang on for days and days. Damn you, bully!

Then, like the hero in every 80's movie, an antioxidant cell comes along and takes away the bully's power. The antioxidant cell creates a stable particle – an allyacne if you will – with the bully, rendering him harmless. Your recovery time improves because your cell regeneration is able to process faster.(ya know, since it's not being picked on by the bully).

However, you can't just smear on some cream that claims to have antioxidants and hope it does the trick – mainly because some of the best and strongest antioxidant particles are too big to penetrate the surface of the skin. If 80's movies taught us anything about bullies, it's that you have to beat them at their own game; you have to neutralize them from the inside.

Adding antioxidant foods is vital to looking amazing on your Big Day so start TODAY by adding one, some, or all of these, into your diet every day: oranges, papayas, kiwi, mango and any red fruits like apples, berries. Good veggies like peppers and sources of beta-carotene like carrots, sweet potatoes and squash; and always get second helpings of green leafy veggies like spinach, kale and romaine lettuce.

Even with a colorful, healthy diet an antioxidant supplement is going to be a great addition to your makeup bag. Later, we'll be doing things to your muscles and skin that are going to need the fast recovery benefit that only antioxidants can provide. A good supplement is a little more viable than just nutritious foods alone because the closer you get to the Big Day, the more stressed out you may get and it will be a lot easier to take a quick vitamin in the morning than it is to run around the kitchen trying to build a colorful fruit salad. Another great reason to start RIGHT NOW!

But remember, a SUPPLIMENT is meant to do just that: SUPPLIMENT your diet. You cannot live on this alone but adding it to your colorful food choices will pay off big time.

When shopping for an antioxidant supplement look for powders vs. pills – your body absorbs the powder faster since it doesn't have to break it down in the stomach. You can find some good options at your drug store or there are several available online and through direct sales. As long as it doesn't have any crazy additives, like caffeine (read the label carefully), then you can take it at night or in the morning. Keep it next to your bathroom sink and think of it as one last step in your skin care routine. Wash your face, take your antioxidant, then do a dramatic fist-pump in the air because you just helped take down the 80's movie free radical bully!

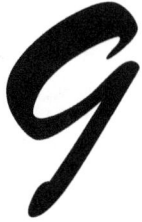

9 WEEKS OUT

9 WEEKS OUT WORKOUT

Pick Up Heavy Things and Put Them Back Down

W hen I see loose skin dangling on the back of the arm on a stranger in the grocery store I want run up and give them a big high-five because I know what it means. It means they have been busting their ass to lose weight and that they probably drag themselves to the treadmill day in and day out, even when they least want to. But I also want to hand them my business card because if we had met at the beginning of their journey, I could have helped them avoid that loose skin or what I call "skinny fat". In the coming weeks, your diet is going to change, your body is going to change and you are going to lose excess fat for your Big Day (yippee!), but to avoid the Bingo Wings that may develop, you have to build up some muscle – which means YOU HAVE TO LIFT WEIGHTS. Unless, of course, your Big Day is a bingo tournament then by all means, skip the muscle building section and let those wings flap with pride!

Last week, your focus was all about choosing your weapons of mass construction, so for your 9-weeks out workout you will be focused on lifting weights. Heavy weights. I know what you're thinking; Doesn't lifting weights make you big? I don't want to get BIGGER! I want lean and sexy arms – not man arms!

First off, you do not have enough testosterone in your body to get ripped like a dude and those men and women train for YEARS to get that look – we only have 9 weeks. Second, you will be getting lean in the coming weeks so your muscles will show through more as the fat cells shrink. Trust me on this one, on your Big Day you do NOT want to raise your pretty, manicured hand to wave and have your bat wing smack some poor, unsuspecting bystander in the forehead.

Plus, during these first few weeks of muscle building, we are actually making your body more metabolically active, which means you'll be burning calories at an accelerated rate. You can burn the same amount of calories in less time with strength training. You've got a Big Day to plan – you can't be spending hours on a dread-mill!

With this week's workout, we designate two body parts per day. This makes the plan easier to follow and in my experience, I find that clients are far more likely to stick with it. If you get your arms done on Monday, you're probably not going to skip Tuesday's leg day or you'll be out of whack and imbalanced.

This also allows ample time to let each muscle group fully recover before you hit it again, giving it the optimal environment to grow. And if you're new to strength training, it means only one part of your body will be tired at a time so you won't feel like your whole body has been put through the ringer.

You have two options: the Print & Go Workout to take to the gym with you or the Print & Stay Workout you can do at home using minimal equipment. You will be using the weights you selected last week. Each day has a single body part in focus so you can mix and match! In case you can't get to the gym you can still do the leg-day moves at home.

Remember, just like Sesame Street, today's workout is brought to you by the number 12 and sponsored by the weight you used last week!

Why 12 reps? According to the National Academy of Sports Medicine, manipulating the muscle to perform each exercise 8-15 times is the optimal way to grow the muscle fiber, or create what's called hypertrophy of the muscle. (NASM Essentials of Personal Fitness Training / Edition 4) It makes the muscle more dense and of course, stronger. And that is exactly what we're trying to do, grow your muscle! We'll work on toning and lengthening later but for right now we build!

Good form is so important when lifting weights so always start with a warm-up set at a lighter weight to make sure you're comfortable with the move. If you're unsure on any of these or don't have access to equipment here is my best trainer advice: GO TO A GYM. Don't feel pressured into buying personal training to get your questions answered, if you see one of the trainers or staff members on the floor ask for help with these moves – it's their job!

Before you head to the club, take a minute to research these moves on YouTube, google and my website (www.kimatthgym.com), it feels great to walk in with a plan and you'll have that "yeah-I-know-what-I'm-doing" air about you. With only one body part in focus per day, you can get in, burn out those muscles and get out within 30-45 minutes.

You can choose to start with exercise #1 and complete 12-16, take a 30-60 rest and then do it again, (three or four times if your schedule allows) or you can do exercise #1, then move to exercise #2, then #3 etc. When you're done with all of them, go back to the beginning and do it again (three or four times if your schedule allows). There is no better way – just do which ever you prefer.

If your week is crunched and you can only get in a few days, choose 2 or 3 exercises from each section and complete your sets and reps as listed. Something is always better than nothing so even if you can only squeeze in 15-20 minutes it will save you from having to squeeze into your big-day outfit!

Print & Stay

Day 1: Leg Circuit

Do this entire list 3 times today. Try 4 if you have time!

1. Bench Step up with Weights
   12 times each leg

2. Weighted Squat on Smith Machine
   12 times

3. Wide Stance Weighted Squat on Smith Machine
   12 times

4. Weighted Walking Lunge
   12 times

5. Single-Leg Lunge with Hop
   30 seconds each leg

6. Leg Press
   12 times

Workout

Do this entire list 3 times today. Try 4 if you have time!

1. Tricep Pull-Down 12 times

2. Bent Rows on Bench 12 times

3. Standing Dumbbell Tricep Extensions 12 times

4. Seated Row 12 times

5. Bench Dips

6. Skull Crushers 12 times

Do this entire list 3 times today. Try 4 if you have time!

1. Dumbbell Bench Press
   12 times

2. Dumbbell Bicep Curls
   12 times each arm

3. Dumbbell Incline Press
   12 times

4. Dumbbell Hammer Curls
   12 times

5. Wide-Position Push-ups
   12 times

6. Concentration Curls
   12 times each arm

7. Chest Fly Machine
   12 times

Day 4: Shoulders and Abs Circuit

Do this entire list 3 times today. Try 4 if you have time!

1. Arnold Press
   12 times

2. Plank
   12 seconds

3. Lateral Raise
   12 times

4. Rear-Delt Raise
   12 times

5. Crunch
   12 times

6. Straight and Oblique Crunches on Ball
   12 each direction - front, left, right

Day 5: Lower-Body Circuit

Do this entire list 3 times today. Try 4 if you have time!

1. Weighted Squats
   12 times

2. Stiff-Legged Deadlift
   12 times

3. Leg Extensions (on machine)
   12 times

4. Hamstring Curls (on machine) or Stability Ball
   12 times

5. Weighted Walking Lunges
   12 times each leg

Day 6: Catch up

Repeat a workout from earlier in the week for whichever body part needs extra attention. Choose muscle groups that will be on display on your Big Day. If you'll be on the beach, spend more time on the legs/tummy. If you'll be wearing a tank or strapless dress, spend the extra time on your upper body.

Day 7: Rest

Print & Stay

Day 1: Leg Circuit

Do this entire list 3 times without rest. Try 4 if you have time!

1. Bench Step Up with Weights

   12 times each leg

2. Weighted Squat

   12 times

3. Weighted Walking Lunge

   12 times each leg

4. Single-Leg Lunge with Hop

   12 times each leg

5. Side Lunge

   12 times each side

Day 2: Back and Triceps Circuit

Do this entire list 3 times without. Try 4 if you have time!

1. Overhead Tricep Extension

   12 times

2. Bent Rows

   12 times each arm

3. Close Grip Tricep Push Ups (if too intense, use wall or chair)

   12 times

4. Bench Dips

   12 times

5. Skull Crushers

   12 times

Day 3: Chest and Biceps Circuit

Do this entire list 3 times without rest. Try 4 if you have time!

1. Dumbbell Press

   12 times

2. Dumbbell Bicep Curls

   12 times each arm

3. Regular Push Ups (if too intense, use wall or chair)

   12 times

4. Dumbbell Hammer Curls

   12 times

5. Wide-Position Push Ups (if too intense, use wall or chair)

   12 times

6. Concentration Curls

   12 times each arm

7. Chest Fly

12 times

Day 4: Shoulders and Abs Circuit

Do this entire list 3 times without rest. Try 4 if you have time!

1. Arnold Press

   12 times

2. Plank with Knee or Leg Raise

   12 each leg

3. Lateral Raise

   12 times

4. Rear-Delt Raise

   12 times

5. Crunch

   12 times

6. Straight & Oblique Crunches on Ball

   12 each direction: front, right, left

Day 5: Lower-Body Circuit

Do this entire list 3 times without rest. Try 4 if you have time!

1. Weighted Squats

   12 times

2. Stiff-Legged Deadlift

   12 times

3. Hip Raises (Lying on Floor)

   12 times

4. Hip Raises (Lying on Side)

   12 times each leg

5. Weighted Walking Lunges

   12 times each leg

Day 6: Catch-Up

Catch Up: Repeat a workout from earlier in the week for whichever body part needs extra attention.

Choose muscle groups that will be on display on your Big Day.

Day 7: Rest

9 WEEKS OUT DIET

It's Time For An Oil Change!

A 2011 study in the New England Journal of Medicine looked at weight gain in a population of 100,000 people. These kind folks had to fill out a diet questionnaire about which foods they ate two or more times per week – ready for a shocker? The people with the most weight gain in a 4 year period, roughly 3.5 pounds per year, all admitted to regularly consuming fried foods. Huh. Who knew?

In case you're not catching onto my sarcasm, stop eating fried foods.

Right now.

In the polish section we discussed what this toxic sludge is doing to your skin but the damage it's doing to the rest of your body is horrific. Cosmetics, cellulite, and muffin-top aside – every batch of fries you eat is increasing your risk of chronic cardiovascular diseases that affect the heart, blood vessels, and brain.

Your pre/post workout meals are still your top priority but integrating the oil change in the Polish section might come as a bit of a struggle so lucky you, that's all you have to focus on this week!

Remember – I don't care about your midnight snack. Nobody is criticizing your 'goody drawer' at work and I don't give a crap about how many calories are in your breakfast. Your only task is focusing on your pre and post workout meals, adding antioxidants to your day and changing your oil. That's it. That's all. Get it done!

9 WEEKS OUT POLISH

Same Oil Change

Hopefully you've integrated last week's polish tip and filled your fridge (and your face) with some power house, antioxidant-rich foods! And with any luck you've also added a good antioxidant supplement and plenty of H20 to your skin care routine. If so, you may already be seeing some small changes. Perhaps a little brighter tone, less redness in areas, probably the dark circles under the eyes are fading. Yippee!

Keep going. It only gets better and better as your dermis (outermost layer of skin) turns over, which can take up to a month. If you haven't yet – GET ON IT! We've only got 9 weeks to go! Antioxidants and hydration are as essential to your make-up bag as mascara!

Comedian Janeane Garofalo said it best when making fun of beauty magazines:

"Headline in a beauty magazine reads 'This summer, a pretty face is your best asset.' Really? As opposed to last summer when back acne and body odor were all the rage?"

Ah, the dreaded back acne, or as I like to call it "bacne." What could be worse on your Big Day? I can't imagine that a big, red shoulder zit goes well with any outfit so let's get to work right now making sure that doesn't happen. Along with your colorful veggies and your new found love for H20, you'll make one teeny-tiny change in your life this week that will change your skin forever: an oil change.

Prep Steps for Your Big Day

I don't imagine you'll be too shocked to hear that cooking with fat or lard is not a common practice for most beauty/ fitness models. Big shocker, I know. But don't be fooled by vegetable or peanut oil either, just because it has the word 'vegetable' in it does not mean it's going to benefit your body. In fact, the harmful effects of these oils on your skin alone are enough reason to leave it on the shelf, not to mention the havoc it's wreaking on your waistline.

So starting today, you are giving your skin an oil change, and it starts by dumping out the vegetable oil. Go to your cupboard right now and dump it out. Go ahead, I'll wait. Don't feel bad about throwing away a whole $2.49 worth of vegetable oil. It's this two dollar and forty nine cent poison that is forcing you to spend hundreds of dollars each year in cleansers, toners and moisturizers! Not only does this stuff clog up your arteries and virtually trap fat in your body but it actually traps bacteria in your skin as well, so no matter how many times you wash your face, those deep-fried whatevers you ate last week are still lurking under your skin, threatening to surface in the form of bacne, chest zits (chits?) and all over breakouts at any moment.

Now that your vegetable oil is in the trash, what will you be cooking with at home? It's simple – replace it will extra virgin olive oil. Anything vegetable oil can do, olive oil can do too but it is so much better for your body and your skin. Use it for sautéing your antioxidant veggies, coating the pan for your eggs, even most baking recipes can be switched out and no one (except your skin and waistline) will know the difference. The switch at home is the easy part. Now comes the hard part. What do you think every restaurant in North America cooks with?

Yep. It's everywhere. Every french fry and onion ring you've ever eaten has been bathed in vegetable or peanut oil. And not even the high-end, expensive, cold-pressed oil. They use the cheapest of the cheap, crappiest of the crap, ruin your skin, kill your dreams of skinny jeans oil.

Of course it is unrealistic to think that you will not be dining out during the next few weeks, as Americans we dine out an average of 3 times a week. Some of my clients turn in their food logs with restaurant bills totaling several hundred dollars a month! But what you eat at those restaurants could literally ruin your Big Day. So be mindful of what you order and stay away from anything fried. That means fries, onion rings, some even batter and fry green beans! Be sure to ask your server how your meat is prepared. That "healthy" chicken salad could be doing a number on your skin.

Easier said than done, I know. Especially when the smells of deep-fat-fried anything comes wafting your way. So here is a very effective habit I get my clients into: when gazing at the menu and your mouth is watering for whatever fried fritters are on special that day, don't say to yourself I can't have that. Because in all honesty, you CAN have that. Of course you can! It's right there, you're paying the bill, you're a grown-ass woman and you can have whatever you want!

But, is that really what you want? Do you want 'bacne'? Do you want to squeeze into spanks? Instead of I can't have that because we all know you CAN, change your words and say (out loud if you have to) I don't want that. Of course you don't! You don't want bacne! You don't want chits! You don't want to spend the next three days popping pimples in your review mirror! You don't want to have to pay to get your zits photo-shopped out of all your Big Day pictures! YOU DON'T WANT THAT!

It's not a matter of will-power. It's not some insane, starve-yourself-stupid diet. It is simply looking at the menu and ordering what you want, and on what could be the big-gest day of your life, you WANT clear skin. So start your oil change right now!

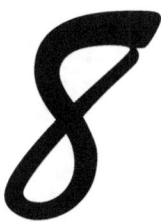

8 WEEKS OUT

8 WEEKS OUT WORKOUT

Keep Picking Up Heavy Things and Putting Them Back Down

Lucky you – no change in your workout this week! We are still focused on building that muscle and changing the shape and tone of your body from the inside out. Your consistency is, by far, the most important thing you can do for your Big Day prep so keep at it!

Continue to lift as heavy as you can for your 12 repetitions and focusing only on one or two body parts per day. It doesn't take long for muscles to develop but in order to keep them, you have to continue to do the work. You will not get 'big' or 'bulky' you're only 2 weeks into a regular lifting program, the super-she-man-muscle-chicks you're so scared of becoming dedicate YEARS in the gym to get that way. 2 weeks doesn't make a she-man.

If you're keeping on track with your pre and post workout meals and of course the uber-important oil change in your diet you will start to notice that your workouts come a little easier this week. Be sure to reward yourself for your dedication – but be careful; do not reward yourself with food- You are not a dog. Download a favorite album from your teen years, treat yourself to a spa day or a massage. Buy yourself a new pair of earrings or some other great accessories for your Big Day.

In the coming weeks we'll be changing up your workout to get you leaner but first we have to get you stronger- keep picking up heavy things and putting them back down!

Happy lifting!

8 WEEKS OUT DIET

How to Build, Shop and
Prepare the Perfect Dinner Plate

We're only a few weeks in and the diet changes have been subtle. Maybe even, dare I say, easy?

Maybe. But maybe not. Cutting the crappy oil out of our ridiculous American diet is sometimes harder than it sounds because it is everywhere! But with only 8 weeks until your Big Day saying 'no thanks' to the greasy stuff should be easier.

You're still focused on your before and after workout meals – fueling up with the really good stuff before like fruits, veggies, and whole grains and the powerful protein afterwards. Those meals have been surrendered to your workouts. And hopefully, when dining out, you're making better choices and going for things that haven't spent some time in the Deep Fat Fryer of Doom.

This week we take over one more of your meals: your dinner plate. I think this is the hardest part for a lot of people. We can do so good with a healthy and lean breakfast, stay on track with healthy snacks and lunches, but when it comes to dinner – its game over. This is when the drive-thru lights call your name or when the cost of the restaurant seems like a better deal than having to dirty up the kitchen. Even easier than having the dreaded "What's for dinner" conversation.

Prep Steps for Your Big Day

I once saw a stand-up comedian who said that when his wife asked him, "What do you want for dinner?" his answer was always the same: "A gun and two bullets so we never have to have this conversation again."

This week, you will learn how to build the perfect dinner on a budget and I'll show you how to do it day in and day out. You'll be less likely to stop by the drive thru and the extra money in your wallet can be put toward your Big Day instead!

Say hello to the list to end all lists. It is the ultimate. In fact, it is literally called The Ultimatest Grocery List, compliments of grocerylists.org, and here's how to use it.

Visit their website (or mine) and print this lifesaver off. On the back write out 5 or 6 meals that you have been craving. Think if I went to a restaurant right now, what would I order? What commercials have you seen lately that looked so good they made your mouth water? What did you smell on the drive home the other day that sounded so delicious?

I have kiddos so I always ask around and see what's on everyone else's palette.

And then there are a few ground rules you need to set for your dinner plate of course:

1) There has to be two handfuls of a vegetable, doesn't matter what kind (although if I were you, I'd make sure they fall into the high-antioxidant category for your skin prep).

2) There must be at least 1 handful of lean protein: chicken, turkey, fish, lean beef, steak, elk, dear, bison, eggs, beans, lean pork, tofu.

3) If your dinner craving is from a restaurant or one of your old-school family fav's, take the time to Printrest

or google a 'clean' recipe for it. It doesn't take a lot of

time to type the word 'clean' before you type the word
'lasagna' and you'll be introduced to a whole new
world of healthy options.

4) If you know you have a late night, be sure to plan
   at least 1 or 2 meals that are quick and easy. It's fun
   to experiment with new recipes but save those for a
   night when you don't have a late meeting or a kiddo's
   soccer practice.

Once you've made your dinner wish list for the week – and
they meet all the criteria listed above – flip over the list and
check the boxes of the things you'll need. Be sure to take a
quick inventory of whatever is already in your fridge so you
don't double up.

Here is another tip: only buy what you need for that week.
Often times, my clients will load up on spinach and broccoli
with all the best intentions of eating it with a shovel day in
and day out, but without a plan, that doesn't happen. The
spin- ach rots before they get to it and they end up throwing
$30 worth of vegetables out and feeling bad about their
squandered intentions.

It does take a minute of planning and a few weeks to get the
hang of it but I have NEVER had a client try this and not love
it. It will change the way you shop, the way you build your
meals, and the way your pants fit!

Why does this work so well? First of all, this list matches the set
up in the store so items that are grouped together in the store are
grouped together on the list. It makes grocery shopping, one of
the devils favorite forms of torture, so much faster and easier.
Plus if you truly do stick to the list, you'll save a ton of money
and since you won't be staring into your fridge wondering what
you can throw together for dinner, your electricity bill may just

shrink a little too!

Secondly, if you have a plan for dinner and it's got the veg-gies, it's got the lean proteins, and it's not cooked in oil, you are on the right track to building healthy meals for the rest of your life as well as not to mention shrinking your waist line for your Big Day. And remember not to get caught up in the Which Veggie Is Better Game. You could have salad, frozen veggies, canned veggies, fresh veggies, steamed veggies, sau-téed veggies (in olive oil of course), it really doesn't matter. Just make sure you've got two handfuls of them on your plate. Also remember; things like canned tomatoes used to make pasta sauces is still a veggie!

I know this may seem archaic. There are 3,000 mobile apps and websites, why can't you just write out your list?

I'll tell you why - there is something magical about this list. Something magical about a pen and a paper and not clicking buttons or spending 30 minutes trying to decipher what my handwriting says. Plus, I forget stuff when I write my own list. When all I have to do is check a box – I am all over it!

When you're done shopping, keep the list of meals up in your kitchen. That way, when someone asks, "What do you want for dinner?" You can answer with "Here are your choices."

This is the same process as all of the online dinner order services that are so popular but way cheaper and you aren't limited to their selections.

Find this list at www.grocerylists.org or at
www.kimatthegym.com to start building your perfect dinner
plate.

The Ultimatest Grocery List! (Compliments of www.grocerylists.org)

FOODSTUFFS

Fresh vegetables
- Asparagus
- Broccoli
- Carrots
- Cauliflower
- Celery
- Corn
- Cucumbers
- Lettuce / Greens
- Mushrooms
- Onions
- Peppers
- Potatoes
- Spinach
- Squash
- Zucchini
- Tomatoes
- ☐
- ☐

Fresh fruits
- Apples
- Avocados
- Bananas
- Berries
- Cherries
- Grapefruit
- Grapes
- Kiwis
- Lemons / Limes
- Melon
- Oranges
- Peaches
- Nectarines
- Pears
- Plums
- ☐

Refrigerated items
- Bagels
- Chip dip
- English muffins
- Eggs / Fake eggs
- Fruit juice
- Hummus
- Ready-bake breads
- Tofu
- Tortillas
- ☐
- ☐

Frozen
- Breakfasts
- Burritos
- Fish sticks
- Ice cream / Sorbet
- Juice concentrate
- Pizza / Pizza Rolls
- Popsicles
- Fries / Tater tots
- TV dinners
- Vegetables
- Veggie burgers

Condiments / Sauces
- BBQ sauce
- Gravy
- Honey
- Hot sauce
- Jam / Jelly / Preserves
- Ketchup / Mustard
- Mayonnaise
- Pasta sauce
- Relish
- Salad dressing
- Salsa
- Soy sauce
- Steak sauce
- Syrup
- Worcestershire sauce
- ☐
- ☐

Various groceries
- Bouillon cubes
- Cereal
- Coffee / Filters
- Instant potatoes
- Lemon / Lime juice
- Mac & cheese
- Olive oil
- Pancake / Waffle mix
- Pasta
- Peanut butter
- Pickles
- Rice
- Tea
- Vegetable oil
- Vinegar
- ☐

Canned foods
- Applesauce
- Baked beans
- Chili
- Fruit
- Olives
- Tinned meats
- Tuna / Chicken
- Soups
- Tomatoes
- Veggies

Spices & herbs
- Basil
- Black pepper
- Cilantro
- Cinnamon
- Garlic
- Ginger
- Mint
- Oregano
- Paprika
- Parsley
- Red pepper
- Salt
- Spice mix
- Vanilla extract

Dairy
- Butter / Margarine
- Cottage cheese
- Half & half
- Milk
- Sour cream
- Whipped cream
- Yogurt
- ☐

Cheese
- Bleu cheese
- Cheddar
- Cottage cheese
- Cream cheese
- Feta
- Goat cheese
- Mozzarella / Provolone
- Parmesan
- Provolone
- Ricotta
- Sandwich slices
- Swiss
- ☐

Meat
- Bacon / Sausage
- Beef
- Chicken
- Ground beef / Turkey
- Ham / Pork
- Hot dogs
- Lunchmeat
- Turkey
- ☐

Seafood
- Catfish
- Crab
- Lobster
- Mussels
- Oysters
- Salmon
- Shrimp
- Tilapia
- Tuna
- ☐

Beverages
- Beer
- Club soda / Tonic
- Champagne
- Gin
- Juice
- Mixers
- Red wine / White wine
- Rum
- Salsa
- Soda pop
- Sports drink
- Whiskey
- Vodka
- ☐

Baked goods
- Bagels / Croissants
- Buns / Rolls
- Cake / Cookies
- Donuts / Pastries
- Fresh bread
- Sliced bread
- Pie! Pie! Pie!
- Pita bread
- ☐

Baking
- Baking powder / Soda
- Bread crumbs
- Cake / Brownie mix
- Cake Icing / Decorations
- Chocolate chips / Cocoa
- Flour
- Shortening
- Sugar
- Sugar substitute
- Yeast
- ☐

Snacks
- Candy / Gum
- Cookies
- Crackers
- Dried fruit
- Granola bars / Mix
- Nuts / Seeds
- Oatmeal
- Popcorn
- Potato / Corn chips
- Pretzels
- ☐

Themed meals
- Burger night
- Chili night
- Pizza night
- Spaghetti night
- Taco night
- Take-out deli food
- ☐

Baby stuff
- Baby food
- Diapers
- Formula
- Lotion
- Baby wash
- Wipes

Pets
- Cat food / Treats
- Cat litter
- Dog food / Treats
- Flea treatment
- Pet shampoo
- ☐

HOUSEHOLD

Personal care
- Antiperspirant / Deodorant
- Bath soap / Hand soap
- Condoms / Other b.c.
- Cosmetics
- Cotton swabs / Balls
- Facial cleanser
- Facial tissue
- Feminine products
- Floss
- Hair gel / Spray
- Lip balm
- Moisturizing lotion
- Mouthwash
- Razors / Shaving cream
- Shampoo / Conditioner
- Sunblock
- Toilet paper
- Toothpaste
- Vitamins / Supplements

Medicine
- Allergy
- Antibiotic
- Antidiarrheal
- Aspirin
- Antacid
- Band-aids / Medical
- Cold / Flu / Sinus
- Pain reliever
- Prescription pick-up

Kitchen
- Aluminum foil
- Napkins
- Non-stick spray
- Paper towels
- Plastic wrap
- Sandwich / Freeze bags
- Wax paper

Cleaning products
- Air freshener
- Bathroom cleaner
- Bleach / Detergent
- Dish / Dishwasher soap
- Garbage bags
- Glass cleaner
- Mop head / Vacuum bags
- Sponges / Scrubbers
- ☐

Office supplies
- CDRs / DVDRs
- Notepad / Envelopes
- Glue / Tape
- Printer paper
- Pens / Pencils
- Postage stamps

Other stuff
- Automotive
- Batteries
- Charcoal / Propane
- Flowers / Greeting card
- Insect repellent
- Light bulbs
- Newspaper / Magazine
- Random impulse buy

Carcinogens
- Arsenic
- Asbestos
- Cigarettes
- Radionuclides
- Vinyl chloride

Other

VODKA MENTOS
MILK
ICE CREAM

IMPORTANT: Please leave this list in the cart when you're done :-)

If found, please mail to Grocerylists.org, P.O. Box 752, St. Louis, MO 63188 USA

Grocerylists.org is the world's largest online collection of found grocery lists. Visit our blog, our hilarious Top 10 lists, check out the book of found shopping lists, or just walk free browsing the thousands of discarded lists in the collection. grocerylists.org.

When you go...
- Take reusable bags!
- Plastic bags to recycle?
- Clip coupons!
- Prepare refill for grill?
- Need to return anything?

Before you check out...
- Need ice?
- Rent a movie?
- Stock up on sale items?
- Use the customer reward card?
- Hand over your coupons!

THE ULTIMATEST GROCERY LIST: THE DELUXE VERSION (V1.1) ©2007-2013 BILL KEAGHY & GROCERYLISTS.ORG.

8 WEEKS OUT POLISH

Moisturize Me!

Radiance is hard to describe. You know it when you see it and you know you want it, but what IS it? Beauty products put it all over their jars and labels and commercials   but it's still a tough nut to crack. Oddly enough, I bet we could make a pretty long list of things we know radiance is NOT:

Bikini line stubble

Arm pit razor burn

Dry, cracked and flaky skin

Self-tanner streaks

As your Big Day gets closer, you'll learn the best ways to tan your skin and the best ways to remove hair. However, from now until then, we've got to prep your skin for what's to come. Along with your water and antioxidants from week 9 and the oil change from last week, there is one crucial skin care step that you have to start this week to be sure the weeks to come are smooth and radiant: MOISTURIZE.

Every time you shower you're stripping away essential oils from your skin. Replenishing with plenty of water intake is a great start (see 10 weeks out polish section) but sealing the deal with a great moisturizer is even better. And you literally are sealing your skin, creating a layer of water-proofing so that all of that beautiful water you've been drinking can stay in your body longer and give your skin better protection from the brutal (but necessary) things you're going to be putting it through in the coming weeks.

What to Use?

First tip is free. Try changing the water temperature in your daily shower to just luke warm. Hot water actually dries you out faster.

Second tip...now that's gonna cost ya! But not much. You don't need to spend hundreds of dollars on a bottle of the fanciest lotion at the specialty beauty store. In fact, since you're going to be using it every single day for the next few weeks, I would suggest you buy the biggest, bulk discount package you can find. And since the active ingredients are the same in most brands – petroleum, beeswax, cocoa butter, olive oil and lanolin – just look for one that you enjoy the fragrance of.

Don't be duped into a separate lotion for each body part, you don't need a separate product for feet than you do for your shoulders. Buy the big bottle and use it everywhere.

The only exception would be your eyes. If you use a face or eye cream it likely has a little different formula so it's safer to use near your eyes without causing irritation.

The trick with moisturizing properly is that there is no trick, just slather it on every time you get out of the shower or bath. Head to toe, every time. Be sure to put plenty on your bikini line and underarm, these areas are the worst to have razor burn and the lotion will help soften the hairs over time, making shaving easier and razor burn less of an issue. Also, be generous on the heels of your feet, knees and elbows. If you go with spray or lotion tan later on, you don't want those areas looking like an orange peel, so start softening them now.

7

7 WEEKS OUT

7 WEEKS OUT WORKOUT

Consistency Trumps Intensity

Hopefully you've enjoyed picking up heavy things and putting them back down. Maybe not the soreness that comes along with it but if your fueling properly on your way to the gym and re-fueling right afterwards, it should be getting more manageable.

We've only got 7 weeks until your Big Day and we're going to make some minor changes to your workouts by shuffling some things around so that you continue to get the lean, sexy look you want for your Big Day.

Week 10 was all about choosing the right weights, weeks 9 and 8 were about putting those weights to work and now with 7 weeks to go, you get to put the weights down for a set. But just one set.

Using your same amount of time at the gym, continue with your same strength training routine but cut the last set of everything and make your way to your favorite cardio equipment. If there is such a thing.

At this stage, we're going to incorporate some low-intensity cardio for a few reasons. First of which is that cardiovascular training burns massive amounts of calories, even when done at a lower intensity. You've already been doing this when you're throwing the weights around but spending a few extra minutes with calorie burning as your main focus will help

prep your heart and lungs and muscle endurance for the weeks to come.

I have great news! You don't need to get blisters on your bum from the spin bike, run until you drip buckets of sweat, or puke, or pass out. There are a lot of workout programs out there that pronounce barfing as the ONLY sign of a good workout. However, there are just as many exercise science studies showing that not only is that level of exertion irrational, it can be down-right dangerous! The key this week is just to get warm and stay there for 15 to 20 minutes every day. At this point, consistency trumps intensity.

So how hard should you work?

Most fitness experts use The Borg Scale of exertion. Developed by Dr. Gunnar Borg, the scale goes from 6 to 20, 6 being the amount of exertion the exerciser feels while doing something very light such as reading a book and 20 being the absolute most energy a person can muster, like the last push at the end of a race. On the Borg Scale 6 relates to a heart rate of roughly 60 beats per minute, an average resting heart rate. The heart rate inclines as the level of work does, up to 20. So 16-20 would equal 160-200 heart beats per minute. Interestingly enough, when participants are given this scale and asked what their perceived exertion is or how hard they think they are working on a scale of 6 to 20, they almost always pinpoint their own heart rates.

Borg was a smart fellow, but a quirky scale of 6 to 20 can be a bit to remember when you have all the numbers of your Big Day fumbling around in your head (number of guests, number of vegetarian guests, cost of XYZ). So I have developed my own, simpler Kim at the Gym scale that I give my clients.

Whether you use this week's Print & Go workout and head to the gym or the Print & Stay workout, just use this simple chart and listen to your body!

Here is my simple 1 to 10 scale of perceived excursion and the thoughts that should be running through your head as you move through these phases of work:

1. Netflix binge day! I'm sitting on this couch until the final credits of the final episode of the final season.

2. I'm enjoying a lovely stroll.

3. Did the heater just turn on? It's warm in here.

4. I'm starting to sweat.

5. I've gotta take this sweatshirt off.

6. Phew! Now I'm movin! I'm so glad I remembered to put on deodorant!

7. Wait...(huff)...Did I..(puff)...put on...deodorant?

8. Words... they are hard.

9. My heart is pounding! My lungs are burning!

10. Oh Dear God, I think I'm going to die!

This week you're only staying around a 5 or 6 so get to know what that feels like. You're warm, maybe taking off your sweatshirt but not feeling like you need to strip down to your sports bra. You're breathing a little more but not panting for air.

Print & Go Cardio

If you're heading to the gym, any cardio equipment will do. As long as it is repetitive and you can maintain it for 15-20 minutes. If you hop on the stair climber, Jacobs' Ladder (the rotating ladder that goes nowhere) or row machine and get to level 8, 9, or 10 in the first 30 seconds, maybe try something else. Those machines are designed to use all your major muscle groups at once and if you're not quite ready for that there is no shame in that game. Just find a piece of equipment that focuses just on legs like a treadmill or bike.

Be warned, those "training zones" or "fat burning" lights and buzzers on the cardio equipment are a total waste of time. Without very specific body testing done by professional trainers or cardiac specialists – like your percentage of body fat, age, blood pressure, cardio vascular condition, resting heart rate - they are completely inaccurate. So just take them for what they are – pretty lights and entertaining noises placed there to sell exercise equipment.

When you do get on a machine, push the Quick Start button every time. You'll get moving quickly (which is the goal) and avoid looking like your trying to read the directions on how to land a Japanese airliner.

If you weren't blessed with "good birthing hips" or have a petite frame, be mindful when you hop on an elliptical. Sometimes the size of these industrial machines build the foot pedals rather widely and the repetitive motion in that awkward stance can cause hip pain or worse problems down the road. So take note to place your feet as closely as possible on the pedals, the very inside edge of the foot cradle.

If you choose a treadmill for your cardio endeavors ….

More power to you! I don't know why I hate that thing so much, it never really did any harm to me, except bore me out of my mind. Maybe it's because it's history is one of torture- in the 1800's they were used to reform prisoners...Not with the intent of getting them healthy – but to torture them for breaking the law! I didn't do anything wrong, why should I have to exercise like I'm in Shawshank?! But it does get the job done, so go ahead. Hit the "quick start" button and off you go. Try not to hold onto the handles as many exercisers end up causing strain to their neck and back by clinging onto the side/front rails for dear life. Plus, that's not really how your body was made to move, swing your arms! You'll burn more calories and actually walk like a human... a human serving life sentence but whatever. If it gets you moving and gets you to a 5 or 6 on the Kim at the Gym scale of exertion – more power to you!

Print & Stay Cardio

One of my favorite memories of my young daughter is when I was in the garage doing a home cardio workout and she asked if she could join me. I only had a few minutes to squeeze in some exercise so I was doing High Intensity Interval Training (HIIT), which you will be learning to love in a few weeks. The workout is 20 seconds of high intensity work followed by a 10 second rest. I happen to have a handy-dandy music download (Tabata, available on iTunes and the App Store) that features a built-in time keeper so I know when my 20 seconds is up.
I told my 6-year-old daughter, "When the coach says go, all you have to do is move your body as much as you can, and when he says stop, you stop and rest."

At the very first interval, the motivating coach voice says "3-2-1 GO!" and my daughter starts flailing about – arms flinging like a windmill, a head jerk and a knee kick every now and then. She looked like she was trying to break out of a straight-jacket while being attacked by bees. When the coach chimes back in 20 seconds later with "3 2 1 Rest" my daughter stops and beams up at me. "Like that, mom? Was that good exercise?"

And you know what? It WAS! She was breathing heavy, and her cheeks were flushed (mine were too, mostly from laughing). But the point is: It doesn't matter how you move your body – you just have to move it!

If you've had a bad day at the office, punch the air and pretend it's your boss for a few minutes. Shovel snow. Take a few trips up and down your stairs. Do jumping jacks. If jumping jacks make you run for the bathroom, take a tip from my 6 year old and just flail about. Just move your body!!!

It drives me crazy when people still cling to the excuse that they don't know what to do at home. Ten years ago I had to write out home programs with things like jumping jacks, run in place, run around the outside of your house, and even I'll admit, those workouts were boring. But now there are so many options! There are countless home DVDs, 300 million fitness YouTubers (some even doing the things from the $40 DVDs) even Netflix and some cable channels have instructional workouts available 24 hours a day!

Of course I own a gym so I am a huge advocate of joining a fitness class with an educated instructor but if you're stuck at home and need to get sweaty (which you absolutely must do if you want to look and feel great on your Big Day) then just move your body. Pretend you just knocked a bee-hive and start moving!

We're 7 weeks out from your Big Day. You still pick up heavy things and put them back down but now, you skip your last set and get a little sweaty. The goal this week is 15-20 minutes, working only at about a 5-6 on my Kim at the Gym scale because, at this point CONSISTENCY TRUMPS INTENSITY.

7 <u>WEEKS OUT</u> DIET

Start a Dairy Diary

W ith only a few weeks to go until you dive into your swim-suit, pose for your photoshoot or rock that dress ,we've got to do a little investigating on what makes you look and feel your best. A few days of observation can lead you to a better understanding of what makes you feel bloated, what makes you pass gas, what makes you feel great and what makes you feel awful. Usually we are so consumed with just getting through our long days we don't take the time to really see what is making our body tick. PS: Could you imagine the embarrassment of passing gas on your Big Day? Just go ahead and let that movie play in your head for a second and then you'll jump right on board with me for this week's prep step.

Most people were raised on milk, yogurt, and cheese and think nothing of it. It "does a body good," right? I remember the celebrity ads with some of my favorite people rocking a milk mustache, (thank you United Dairy Council for your fine advertisements on my young impressionable mind) but it wasn't until I really started scrutinizing my intake that I realized how bloated I was after that ice-cream, latte or yogurt.

Every BODY is different and responds to the proteins and enzymes of dairy differently. It may depend on what you were raised eating, or whether you were breast-fed, or how the diary is processed. But let's say the morning of your Big Day you are in a blind test and you know that the drink in Cup A

is going to make you a fart, possibly at the most inopportune time, and the drink in Cup B won't. Which one would you choose?

So now we need to find out how the ingredients in Cup A really affect you. Let's start by a simple switch-a-roo. All you have to do this week is drop your dairy and replace it with almond, soy or rice milk. The cost is close to the same at the grocery store and it's an easy switch for the barista at the coffee shop. Anything you might cook using milk can be replaced as well. Also, stay away from any yogurt and cheese this week – I know easier said than done but it's in the name of research!

Making the switch is the easy part, the challenge comes from really observing what differences you feel and that's where the diary helps. You may not realize how bad you feel right now since you haven't ever been to the "other side" or you may not notice a difference at all. But journaling will help you make the connection. It doesn't have to be fancy, a simple paper pad or note app on your phone will help you remember the cause and effect of the dairy you ate.

Look for things like bloating, an increase or decrease in gas, headaches coming or going away, tummy cramps when using the restroom. Also, be mindful to see if you feel like you have brain fog or more energy. After a few days you might even notice that your joints feel better/worse and that may be due to inflammation that is sometimes caused by dairy.

The notes can be simple. It's just a way to remind you what you tried and how it affected you, for example:

Day 1 — No dairy today. Feel fine.

Day 2 — No dairy. Tried soy milk latte. GASSY! My dog won't sit by me.

Day 3 — No dairy. Tried Almond Milk in my latte. Dog came back.

Day 4 — No dairy for 4 days, no headache for 3 days

Day 5 — Almond milk, good on cereal. Jeans fit looser today?

Day 6 — Ate some cheese = cut some cheese

Day 7 — When will this prep-step be over? I want ice-cream!

Once you have a clear understanding of how dairy affects you and you venture out to find some alternatives it's like a whole new grocery store opens up to you. You can find tons of yogurts and frozen desserts made from rice, soy, coconut or almond milks.

Then again, dairy may not have any negative effects on you at all. But wouldn't you rather know for sure so that you're not backstage on your Big Day slamming Gas-X®?

7 WEEKS OUT POLISH

Schlep It Off

Your skin has been at this for 3 weeks now, which should be ample time for the dermis to turnover (usually 20-30 days, depending on age). We've drenched it inside and out by increasing your water intake and moisturizing after every shower/bath. Plus, the antioxidant supplementation has increased production of your new, healthier cells. When it's time for the stronger new cells to make an appearance, the old, dead cells falls off on their own but sometimes those little buggers hold on way longer than they need to, making your complexion look dull and dry. They can even clog your pores and cause acne and blemishes.

We've only got 7 weeks until your Big Day, we don't have time for any damage-causing cling-ons! It's time to schlep off the old to make room for the new.

This week you'll be adding a new skin regime in your shower, a magical little routine to remove dead skin cells and help the new, healthy ones to surface even faster.

Exfoliation!

Oh, you've heard of it? Great! Go do it!

You can use a store-bought exfoliating body or face wash which usually have small sugar crystals, or seeds, to give the abrasiveness we need, or find a regular liquid wash and use

Prep Steps for Your Big Day

a loofa/rough sponge to scrub your body. Be sure to change your loofa regularly as those tend to hold onto bacteria and you may consider using a smaller, less abrasive sponge for your face.

Another option is to make your own scrub with some stuff you probably already have in your kitchen. Oatmeal works great for sensitive skin and pure sugar crystals mixed with your favorite smelling oil works great too.

Remember the idea is to scrub off the dead layer of skin so a little pressure is good. Aggressively scrapping your skin till you bleed, is not. A gentle exfoliation will do the trick and since this will be part of your daily routine now, a gentle scrub everyday will help get rid of the cling-ons and make room for your new cells to shine.

Exfoliating is strictly a pre-shave event. It helps to raise the hair so shaving is easier but you need to rinse off completely before applying your shave gel to avoid an uneven or bumpy path for your razor. And remember to never scrub your freshly shaved skin with an exfoliator... Ouch.

This step is crucial right now as we prep your skin for your tan, hair removal and makeup. Your dermis layer will still turn over a few more times before your Big Day, and since you're going to continue to drink plenty of water, take your antioxidants, exfoliate and moisturize you are sure to have a fresh, clean, flawless pallet to work with. Any makeup artist will tell you that will make all the difference!

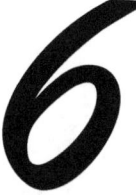

6 WEEKS OUT

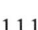

6 WEEKS OUT WORKOUT

Living Well is the Best Revenge

Oddly enough I write this chapter exactly 6 weeks out from the photo shoot for the cover of this book and so, dear reader, from here on out, we are in this together! Most of the stuff you've read so far, I do regularly and hopefully you've seen such incredible changes in your body, energy, and skin that you're going to integrate them for the rest of your life as well. But for these last two months, (OMG! You have less than two months until the Big Day!) we're going to get laser focused. For this week's prep step we need to dial in on exactly what YOU need to focus on for your Big Day. The workouts this week really depend on what you'll be wearing or what you'll be doing on your Big Day.

I have helped clients prep for all kinds of things and it is imperative that we start now to develop the muscles that you know you'll be using (or showing off) on your Big Day. It could mean the difference between a horrible vacation and a great one! For example, if you're prepping for a vacation and you'll be zip-lining through the Costa Rican rain forest, you should probably take some time to develop your upper-body strength so the Toucans don't poop on you while you dangle from the line, arms spent, and waiting for the guide to come get you. If your Big Day is meeting with some old friends for a week of water skiing or hiking, then building up some endurance in your legs will save you from wasting two days of your vacation on the couch whining about how sore you are.

113

Functionality of the muscle is important and it takes time, but let's face it, sometimes your only goal is to look smoking hot and that takes time too. Obviously, I knew what I was going to be wearing for this book cover so I needed to spend this time on my shoulders, arms, chest and back.

Let's say you're 8 weeks out prepping for your high-school reunion. A cocktail dress is perfectly appropriate and may expose your chest, calves and arms so we can pay special focus developing those areas, without neglecting the rest of your body. Plus, when you combine these workouts with the polish techniques you will look like you've been living a healthy lifestyle for years – and I don't care where you went to high school there is always someone there you can't wait to stick it to. As they say, living well is the best revenge. (Insert evil laugh). So let's make it look like you've been living well for a long, long time. Ha!

Think for a moment about what you'll be wearing or what you'll be doing. You may not know exactly what your full ensemble will be but by now, with only a few weeks to go, you're sure to have some vague idea.

To increase your endurance and really focus on developing each muscle (without neglecting the rest of the body) we're going to add in Super Sets this week. Or as I like to call them Super-Duper Sets!

This is where we do two exercises back to back with no rest. This will increase your intensity which will raise your heart rate and burn some extra butter. It fatigues the muscle faster so we're doing fewer exercises. You may even notice your gym/workout time is a little less than usual, which is a good thing! It means you are getting stronger as your body muscle is getting used to the workouts you've been doing. This is the perfect time to switch it up! Continue to fuel your workout well and eat correctly when you're done.

Print & Go

Super Sets For Super Muscles

Day 1: Leg Circuit

Do this entire list 3 times today.
Then move to low intensity cardio.

1. Bench Step Up With Weights — NO REST

   12 times each leg

   add 12 Jump Squats, then rest

2. Weighted Squat – NO REST

   12 times

   add 12 Fast Body Weight Only Squats, then rest

3. Weighted Walking Lunge — NO REST

   12 times

   add 12 Jumping Lunges, then rest

Day 2: Back and Triceps Circuit

Do this entire list 3 times today.
Then move to low intensity cardio.

1. Tricep Pull-Downs — NO REST

   12 times

   add 12 Bench Dips, then rest

2. Lat Pull Down — NO REST

   12 times

   add 12 Bent Barbell Rows, then rest

3. Laying Dumbbell Triceps Extension (skull crushers) — NO REST

   12 times

   add 12 Standing Triceps extensions, then rest

Day 3: Chest and Biceps Circuit

Do this entire list 3 times today.
Then move to low intensity cardio.

1. Dumbbell Bench Press – NO REST

   12 times

   add 12 Fast Push-ups, then rest

2. Dumbbell Bicep Curls – NO REST

   12 times

   drop weight and add 12 lighter curls, then rest

3. Chest Fly Machine- NO REST

   12 times

   add 12 Wide Push Ups, then rest

Day 4: Shoulders and Abs Circuit

Do this entire list 3 times today.
Then move to low intensity cardio.

1. Plank – NO REST

   30 seconds

   add 12 down dog pushups, then rest

2. Lateral Raise- NO REST

   add 12 Front Raises, then rest

3. Over Head Press – NO REST

   add 30 seconds of speed bag (Just like it sounds,
   pretend you are hitting a speed bag over your head,
   circling fist over fist)

4. Hold Right Side Plank 30 seconds- NO REST

   lie on back and add 20 right side crunches

5. Hold Left Side Plank 30 Seconds – NO REST

   lie on back and add 20 left side crunches

Day 5: Lower-Body Circuit

Do this entire list 3 times today.
Then move to low intensity cardio.

1. Weighted Squats – NO REST

   12 times

   add 12 Jump Squats (no weight)

2. Stiff-Legged Deadlift – NO REST

   12 times

   add long stance walking lunge, stepping out as far as you can

3. Leg Extensions (on machine)- NO REST

   12 times

   add 12 Body Weight Squats

Day 6: Low Intensity Cardio

Day 7: Rest

6 WEEKS OUT DIET

Breaking Bread

Remember, as I write this, I am weeks out from my own Big Day, the photo shoot for the cover of this book. Which, with any luck, will infiltrate the front tables and windows of every bookstore in America. I try to maintain fairly clean eating (but far from spotless) and a consistent workout routine for my health (and sanity), but trust me, I do not live and breathe fitness like some of my gym cronies. Don't get me wrong, I'd love to, but most of my time is consumed by raising my kids, paying my mortgage and getting other people to their goals. I really only shift my focus to myself when I have something big coming. This photo shoot will be one of my Big Days and good or bad, in this industry, I have a lot of them. There is a lot riding on these pictures since they will be used on most of my media outlets, my webpage and of course this book. So clearly, back-fat is not an option.

These past few weeks have been general fitness and wellness tips that are always part of my program and hopefully, you've seen enough positive changes that they will be part of your wellness from now on. Refrain from fried foods, keep your water and antioxidant intake high, and use your dairy diary to know how certain foods affect you. For the next 6 weeks, everything you read is on point with what fitness models and industry experts know as the "cutting" secrets to looking your best, leanest self. I hope you take comfort in the fact that I'll be doing it right along with you. And when my next photo shoot, speaking engagement, reunion comes up I will do it again just like you

Prep Steps for Your Big Day

Starting this week we (you and me) are cutting out BREAD. I know it sucks. But read this again, we are cutting out BREAD, not carbs. Remember there are lots of great carbs out there and you're going to need them for your workouts so do not confuse this for one of those no carb diets. This is a simple drop or, in some cases, a simple switch to ensure you look lean and strong for your Big Day.

Don't panic, this isn't for the rest of your life. And don't be mad – up to this point, I haven't asked you cut anything out of your diet except your oil change and dairy that makes you gassy- so let's stay friends. You and Sara Lee® will meet again, but for the next 6 weeks, we're going to drop the dinner rolls, skip the toast, say "No, thank you" to the bagels, and cross off the croissants. The reason for this bread cut is HUGE and it will make a big impact on how you look and feel on your Big Day.

First off, it's an obvious calorie cut, especially if bread is a staple with your breakfast or on your dinner plate. This simple drop could cut hundreds of needless calories out of your day and you'll see a dramatic drop on the scale.

But the question is, if Dave's Killer Breads® are no longer on the sandwich menu, what's going to hold your turkey? And if toast isn't an option on the breakfast menu, what will I eat with my eggs?

For your multiple questions, your answer is multiple choice:

  a) Go shopping.

  b) Substitute with a veggie.

  c) Do without.

Option A) Go Shopping.

By this I mean it's time to hit your local natural grocer and look for an interesting and healthy wrap, tortilla, or pita. When you really start exploring other turkey holder options, you'll be amazed at what's available. There is some sort of bread-like product in every culture and most (if not all) are better for you than traditional American-style bleached-flour-based breads. So get to the store or hop online and start shopping! Look for things with very few ingredients and no preservatives. Remember to eat it quickly (within a few days), because foods with no preservatives are great to nourish your body but they aren't made to last, unlike our American breads that have a longer shelf-life than I do. Also, try to incorporate the lesson from Week 10 and make sure the very first word in the ingredient list is "whole." You'll also want to keep these types of carbs limited to early in the day. I'm going to write that again for dramatic effect and also to make sure you get it: limit breads (no matter how healthy they are) to early in the day.

Option B) Substitute with a veggie.

What? You've never heard of a lettuce wrap? If you're just looking for something to hold your tuna fish, any kind of lettuce works great. It costs about a dollar for a head, gives a little crunch and adds zero calories. This substitution rule also works for that empty void on your dinner plate where your flaky roll used to be. Fill that blank space with a second helping of your veggies or another veggie all together. Don't over think it or dirty a new pan to create the next Wolfgang Puck side dish. Just toss a few carrots, sugar snap peas, or cucumbers in the blank space. Any veggies, prepared any way you like, (except deep-fat-fried, of course).

Option C) Go without.

Does this one really need an explanation? I know it sucks. Dinner rolls are yummy. Donuts are freaking delicious. But we are trying to get RID of rolls remember! Fear not, you will taste them again, but until your Big Day, we're going to pass the bread basket with our heads held high

6 WEEKS OUT POLISH

The Best-kept Hair Secret Ever in the History of Ever

I am a bit of a hair product hog. My shower is lined with hair care products from every corner of the salon. The bathtub is surrounded with bottles promising to thicken, lengthen, strengthen, curl and smooth. I am not brand-loyal so I buy whatever is on special, whoever has the prettiest bottle and if the label touts some unknown, exotic ingredient, I'm all over it.

Krypto-Hydro-Karatene-Beta-Alpha-Complex?! Yes, please! Just what my hair has always needed!

Hair care marketing companies LOVE me. I will buy the cheapest wash-and-toss underwear or the off-off-brand dish soap at the not-even-a-dollar store but when it comes to hair products I will spend. I buy new shampoo and conditioner often with the justification that I haven't found the "right one" yet. Being a trainer, I sweat a lot so I wash my hair often and I am constantly pulling it back or piling it into a bun, causing damage and breakage. So shelling out fistfuls of money for the "right one" would be worth every penny to me. I buy small sizes from high-end beauty stores or salons and use them for a week or so, maybe a month, and then I'm on to the next. The space under my sink is where the half-used bottles go to die. Or into my daughter's shower. But when the product graveyard started getting too full (according to my husband, not me) I had to do something.

131

Prep Steps for Your Big Day

So I asked my stylist, and dear friend, for a solution to be sure I would have the best looking hair on my Big Day (the photo shoot for this book). And sure enough, she gave me a literal solution:

2 tablespoons of Dawn dish soap (3 tbsp. for longer hair)

+

2 tablespoons of Baking Soda (3 tbsp. for longer hair)

Mix together in a small bowl and massage into scalp and hair just like shampoo, let sit for 3-5 minutes and rinse. Immediately follow with a high-quality repairing shampoo & conditioner from a salon or beauty supply store – not the grocery store.

I will warn you, when you rinse this concoction out your hair will feel like straw. Worse, actually, your hair will feel like wet straw. It doesn't give your hair that soft, silky, run-your-fingers-through-it feeling because it is actually stripping old residue off of your hair. It turns out that even the priciest of pricy hair care products leave a residue on your hair all the way from your scalp to the tip. We build up this goopy scum with every single wash, every sprits of hairspray, every dab of argon oil – no matter how fancy the product is, it is piling up on each strand! The sodium bicarbonate (baking soda) is sometimes used in hair care products but it's usually diluted with all kinds of other foo-foo stuff to make it smell and look good.

By using this active ingredient raw, the small crystals of the substance give each follicle a little scrub down, just like when you exfoliate your skin. The dish soap, as you may know from commercials, cuts through grease and oil.

I thought her idea for baking soda and dish soap was absolutely crazy, especially when you first rinse it out and your tresses feel like swamp weeds. But, when you go back in with a high-quality shampoo and conditioner (it doesn't even matter what brand) you'll add back some of that moisture without the buildup and your hair will feel A-MAZE-ING!

When I started telling my clients about this, one of them in the beauty industry said, "Oh, yeah, I wash with baking soda a couple times a year." WHAT!? Beauty experts have known this for YEARS and I am just now finding out?! I felt betrayed. What about the $7,000-worth of hair products in my shower? I could have spent $1.50 on a box of Arm & Hammer® years ago and saved myself some anguish and shelf space.

You can do this trick every 6 weeks or so if necessary to remove product build-up but don't be tempted to do it too often as it can upset the pH balance of your hair and cause breakage.

So there you go, you are 6 weeks out from your Big Day and that is your polish assignment for the week. Go dig for the orange box in your baking cupboard and get to cleansing. Whether you decide to color your hair, curl it, cut it or leave your locks flowing, this step will cleanse and prep your hair and make it much for manageable for whatever style you decide on for your Big Day.

Prep Steps for Your Big Day

5

5 WEEKS OUT

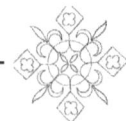

5 WEEKS OUT WORKOUT

Gotta Take Your HIITs

Aright, the consistency is there, the work is getting done and the changes are happening! Now, with 5 weeks until the Big Day it's time to up your calorie burn.

In his film Fat, Sick, and Nearly Dead, Producer Joe Cross asked strangers on the street the burning question: "What is a calorie?" Their answers were shocking! People said things like, "I don't know what they are, but I know their bad for you."

Sadly, most people have been misinformed about calories and what they truly are so I hope this chapter helps clear some things up for you. First off, to measure something in calories is simply a measurement of energy – just like an inch is a measurement of length, or a pound is a measurement of weight.

So if you have 400 calories, you have 400 units of energy.

Your workouts so far have been expending some energy for sure, lifting weights requires energy output, Super-Duper-Sets require energy output, but your cardio prescription has been fairly minimal as you've been instructed to stay in the 5 to 6 range on the scale. Still an energy output but by now your body is capable of more.

Prep Steps for Your Big Day

This week, we're going to up that energy output to its absolute max! But only in short bursts.

HIIT or High Intensity Interval Training is not a new concept, most professional athletes in the NFL and NBA, even hockey players do this style of training because that is what the game requires. To adopt the physiologic benefits for the average person, someone had to put a name to it (HIIT) and some guidelines.

Basically, HIIT workouts use your body's ability to push incredibly hard for short bursts of time. We all have this handy superpower of being able to run at amazing speeds in the event of a bear chasing us. But sadly, we aren't built to sustain that type of exertion for very long. This superpower is fueled by your body's ability to produce ATP (or Adenosine Triphosphate) and it will fuel your body at any time to give you a massive burst of energy. Catch is, it can only last about 2 minutes. After roughly 2 minutes, your body changes gas tanks and begins using other fuel sources like carbohydrates, fat, and even muscle.

The theory with these high intensity intervals (which has been proven in several studies by the University of North Carolina and the American College of Sports Medicine) is that your body's need for oxygen during the effort will create an oxygen shortage, thus during the recovery or rest periods, your body has to ask for more oxygen which leads to burning more calories. So you get this incredible "after burn" that you don't get from steady-state exercise, or exercise where your heart rate stays the same for long time.

So you can do 20 minutes of steady cardio, where your heart rate goes up and stays up and you burn a moderate amount of calories. Or you can do 20 minutes of HIIT exercises where the heart rate goes up and down and you'll burn more calories when YOU'RE DONE exercising. It's like the gift that keeps on giving! The workout that lasts all day! Yippee!

So let's HIIT it!

When it comes to HIIT training the focus should be on the H and the I – as in HIGH INTENSITY. Where your last workout had you maintain a 5 or a 6 on the Kim at the Gym scale and you maybe got warm enough to take your outer layer off, this time we want to push you more to a 7 or 8, maybe even a 9! (Remember, 10 means call the paramedics so please don't get there.) Your heart should be pounding. You should be open-mouth breathing. Your lungs should be pissed. You should be questioning why you started this in the first place! And you should definitely be stripping off your layers of clothes. But the good news is, you only have to feel like that for a short burst. A very short burst. About 20-30 seconds at max.

Just when you think you cannot maintain that intensity for one more second, you rest and take a 10 second break. 10 seconds doesn't seem like a very long time and you're right, it's not. But it is enough time to catch your breath, give yourself a little pep-talk, and maybe even snap a selfie before you get back to your intense interval.

Since we only have 5 weeks to go, now is the time to push your caloric burn to the max and get into jaw-dropping shape for your Big Day!

Here are some of the best interval moves to try in your routine, and remember it is MAX intensity or else the entire concept is pointless. It's not called Moderate Intensity Interval Training (MIIT? Lame.)

So don't hold back on any of these! Give them all you've got, push harder than you think you can. It's only 30 seconds! You can do anything for 30 seconds!

- Jumping Lunges

- Jumping Sumo Squats

- Mountain Climbers

- Burpees

- Star Jumps

- Tuck Jumps

- Sprint Runs

- High Knee Run in place

- Fast Feet

- Puddle Jumps

- Side to Side (Ice Skaters) for distance

- Side to Side Ice Skater for speed

- Speed Squats

- Butt Kickers

- Wide Stance High Knee Run in place

Prep Steps for Your Big Day

Take this list and go through the moves at full force for 30 seconds. Take a 10 second rest in between each move, or try each move for 2 sets each so your workout would look like this:

High Knee Run in place (30 Seconds)

Rest (10 seconds)

High Knee Run in place (30 Seconds)

Rest (10)

Next move

If none of this sounds appealing, just take a page from my daughter's book and flail about through space, as long as it's your max output. Remember your thoughts are not "Gee, golly gosh. I'm getting a bit warm." But more like "Oh Dear God!! My lungs are fire!!!!" If you're a gym-goer you can certainly get this done on your favorite piece of cardio equipment. It really doesn't matter if you choose to move at peak speed on a machine like a stationary bike or elliptical, just move! Remember, your maximum output for 30 seconds.

Use your phone as a timer or watch the second hand on a clock and push hard. When your 10 second rest comes, be mindful to take long, deep breaths to calm the heart rate as quickly as possible. A simple trick is to breathe in through your nose and out through your mouth as the nasal cavity will warm the air before it hits your lungs and make the distribution work a little easier for the cardio-respiratory system.

There are also some songs and timers available on iTunes or your favorite music stations. Just search "Tabata" on your device, and go!

And then rest for 10 seconds and go again!

5 WEEKS OUT DIET

Finding the Sugar Boogers

W ith only 5 weeks to go until you're walking down the aisle, stepping off the plane, or meeting that special someone, it's time we tackle the hardest part of the program. In fact, this can be so tough for some people we're going to spend the next two weeks focusing on just this point. Brace yourself... it's time to wrangle in your sugar intake.

Sugars are just like little boogers because they hide. Everywhere. Even with all the changes you've made so far by adding all of those wonderful, colorful fruits and veggies into your day; even when your pre and post-workout meals are dialed in and you know exactly what your dinner plate is going to look like; even though you've cut a majority of the bread products out of your day and you've learned which dairy or non-dairy products work best to avoid bloating; even with all of these amazing healthy changes you may be surprised at just how much sugar you ingest every day.

In the next section, you'll learn more about why sugars are such boogers but for now, let's just figure out what kind of a beast we need to battle.

We'll kick off this week by taking a sugar inventory. Remember we're just recording, not changing anything... Yet.

If you can't see it, you can't fix it, so get out your magnifying glass because even though your intake of the obvious sugar sources like your lattes and desserts may be shocking, when you discover how many hidden sugars you're eating in a day it may just blow your mind!

Your cereal box may say 12 grams but did you add the milk sugars? That granola bar may rock the whole grains and have substantial protein, but the sugars may be enough to send your insulin levels into a tailspin. Your coffee creamer, ketchup, salad dressings, drinks – it all adds up! So, just like the dairy diary, I'll ask you spend this week totaling up your daily sugar intake. Remember it doesn't have to be fancy, and – bonus - you don't even have to count sugars found in your fruits/ veggies.

Here are a few tips to help you track:

1) Be sure to check the label on EVERYTHING that has a label but don't get caught up in hunting down the sugar content in natural foods like apples, strawberries etc.- (You know, the colorful foods you've been eating for the high antioxidants).

2) Be truthful in your serving size. For example, if the caramel syrup label in your mocha says the serving size (20g) is 1 tbsp. and the barista slams 3 pumps into your cup, that is closer to 3 tbsp. So you better multiply that 20g of sugar by 3 equaling 60 grams.

3) This week is only a fact-finding mission. We can't fix what we can't see, so don't worry about good/bad just track how much sugar goes into your mouth in a day.

4) Don't be oblivious to the obvious. Clearly the chocolate cake after dinner, the cookies in the break room, the sweet treats in the candy dish are sources of sugar so WRITE THEM DOWN.

5) Don't be oblivious to the not-so-obvious. Check the labels on your salad dressings, dipping sauces, drinks, snacks, and coffee creamers.

Example:

Day   Approx. Sugar Totals

Monday — 200 grams (Office B-day Cake)

Tuesday — 60 grams

Wednesday — 160 grams (Drive-through coffee)

Thursday — 90 grams

Friday — 300 grams (Dined out)

Saturday — 200 grams (Movies)

Sunday — 300 grams (Family BBQ)

5 WEEKS OUT POLISH

Wax vs. Sugar vs. Shaving

With only a few weeks out until your Big Day we have to think about how we want to tame the beast of burden that is our body hair. I know it seems silly to put it on your priority list with so much time until your Big Day but it really depends on which route you go to remove your fur coat. Every body's hair is a little different and grows at different speeds, thickness, and texture and there are tons of ways to remove it. In your everyday life you may have a great routine but for something as special as your Big Day you want to be stubble free but still allow time for any irritation to subside.
With all the different options, you may even want to try a new method, but how do you prep and how do you choose? Allow me to shed some light on how to remove hair from the places where the sun don't shine.

If you've followed the tips from previous chapters by hydrating, taking a daily anti-oxidant, exfoliating, and moisturizing every day, then you've already done most of the leg work to ensure smooth skin (pun intended) and now you just need to decide how you want to remove the hair. Here are few of the best prep tips and timing guidelines for whichever method you choose:

Shaving:

One of the nice benefits of this method is that your grow-out length doesn't have to be substantial and you don't need to worry about booking an appointment. But with so much time to spare, it is a good time to start experimenting with different brands of blades. Some think that all blades are the same whether it costs $1.00 or $12 and for the most part, it's true. Who hasn't borrowed a men's razor in a pinch? It still gets the job done. But what's unique to different brands is the shape of the handle, the number of blades, and maybe a lubricating strip. So it's nice to have time to test drive a few so you can find one that works well for you. When it comes time for the final Big Day shave though, be sure to use a BRAND NEW razor. They are called disposable razors for a reason, they aren't meant to be used for months and months as those little blades can house a lot of bacteria that can cause nasty out breaks, ingrown hairs, and infections.

Timing: If you're prone to razor burn I would advise that you allow for at least 3-5 days of growth before your Big Day shave and consider blocking some time the night before, just in case you do get a little cut, you don't bleed on your Big Day outfit and any irritated skin can have time to heal. If you have to shave on the day of, prevent razor burn by splashing with cold water on your skin immediately after shaving. And if those little red bumps do pop up, try a cold compress by putting a few ice cubes in a thin towel and hold on the irritate area for about 5-10 minutes. It soothes the area and will reduce inflammation – and remember, if your antioxidant intake is high- that will help.

And one last tip on shaving for your Big Day, use only luke warm water in your bath or shower, hot water will swell the skin so you're not getting as close of a shave as you may think.

True Story of waxing vs. sugaring:

In researching for this book, I called around to several local spas for prices and information and settled on a mid-range salon that was a bit of a drive from my house (they had the nicest receptionist). I asked the consultant if I could have waxing done one side of my bikini line and sugaring done on the other so I could compare the whole process, the pain level, the grow out etc.
What I share with you now are the findings from said mission...

Waxing:

If this is the route you want to go, then you want to start... um... "Growing your garden" right now. In order for the wax to adhere, the hair needs to be AT LEAST as long as a grain of rice. Depending on how fast or slow your hair grows, this can take weeks. It is true that the more often you wax, the less you have to do it but that takes several treatments as your hair will need to go through a few growth cycles and be pulled out by the follicle.

Waxing can be a bit pricy ($30-$200 depending on where you live and how much area you want deforested) but your smooth skin can last about 7-10 days before you start to see any stubble so if your Big Day involves a lot of beach time, this may be the route you choose.

If you've never had the pleasure of having your hair ripped out by the root, let me enlighten you. The process involves an appointment with an esthetician (yes, you must go to a professional) at least the first few times to learn the timing and techniques and avoid making a goopy mess in your bathroom.

The sweet and friendly beautician will apply a bit of baby powder to your nether regions (to absorb moisture) while you tell them all about your Big Day. You'll think, "This is nice, it's great to get pampered like a baby." Next, she will apply warm wax with a stick or spatula. This part is nice too. Soothing.

You'll continue to make small talk with your pleasant new friend while the wax is left to cool on your skin for 20 or 30 seconds so it dries around the hair. You'll think "Gee, this isn't so bad. Besides having my lady business on parade, I feel completely comfortable with this person. It's nice to have a pal in the beauty business."

But then, the esthetician, who seemed charming and calm at first, suddenly channels all of their rage and regret into their fingertips and with one mighty jerk, she rips the dried wax off as fast and as hard as she can! It will seem as though this small, pretty person has channeled ridiculous amounts of strength from Satan himself.

It sucks the first time. It hurts the first time. And anyone who says it doesn't is lying.

But it only hurts for a second. Your ex-bestie will immediately apply pressure and move on to the next area before you have time to run and slash her tires. The whole event is very quick and a little anticlimactic, since it took you so long to grow that fur and then it goes away so quickly you barely have time to say goodbye.

If you choose to wax there are a few tricks to make it a little less awful. First of which is one you should be doing already – exfoliating! Removing the dead cells from the skin and any residue built-up on the hair will help the wax adhere better and the whole thing will go much smoother. Ha! Get it?

Next, you could go to a beauty supply store before your appointment and look for a numbing cream. This needs to be applied about 30-45 minutes before the waxing to be effective so most spas don't offer it since you'd have to sit in their treatment room taking up valuable spa real estate. But it's an easy thing to do on your own and may make the whole experience more pleasurable. Also, a shot of your favorite adult beverage before your appointment couldn't hurt.

Timing: You may have a little irritation that looks like razor burn after your first session but it doesn't last long and, as I said, the results do last long enough to enjoy a full week on the beach so I would book your waxing appointment for 2-3 days before your Big Day. You'll stay smooth for your entire vacation and still allow time for irritation to subside.

Grow out: The waxing did irritate my skin a little as it was my first time with this sort of torture. But the small bumps that looked like razor burn went away within a day or two and my skin was silky smooth for about a week. I did have to dig out the razor for an occasional rogue hair spiking up, but the effort was minimal compared to having to contort myself into impossible positions to shave every other day.

The other bummer is the grow-out length. In order to go back for another waxing you've got to commit to that grain-of-rice-grow-out-length which means you've got to power through the I-Don't-Care-If-I'm-In-Public-I-Have-To-Itch-My-Business phase and the Oh-My-God-Don't-Touch-Me-I-Look-Like-A-Wooly-Mammoth phase before you can book your next session.

Sugaring:

Sugaring for hair removal is not a new thing. It was actually invented in ancient Egypt and is sort of making a comeback in the beauty scene. The concept is very similar to waxing but instead of wax, that can be made of harmful chemicals, the specially-trained esthetician applies a concoction made primarily of sugar, a more earth friendly choice. It's not as warm as the wax, just a sugary goop that smells nice and then a piece of thin paper is placed on top and acts like tape to stick to the sugar. As with the waxing, one good pull is all it takes to rip the hair out. But here's the kicker: because the sugar doesn't adhere to the hair as much as the cooling wax does your beauty buddy may have to go over the same spot a few times. So there you have it, nature girl. If you want to enjoy that thrashing in the same spot over and over again, be my guest. It may be better for the earth but my mother nature did NOT enjoy it.

Grow out: With the sugaring, there were certainly less razor burn-like bumps so my skin looked a lot better on the day of and the day after. However, the grow-out within a few days was almost identical. A few rogue hairs, about a week's worth of silky smoothness and then it was back to the razor for me.

I only gave it one attempt in the name of research so I can't attest to what might happen after 3 or 4 treatments (my next book perhaps?) but for your Big Day you may find that it's worth it to splurge on a little spa pampering. Or skip the whole painful thing and spend that money on a massage! You'll be so relaxed, you won't mind how hairy you are!

Prep Steps for Your Big Day

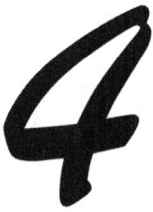

4 WEEKS OUT

4 WEEKS OUT WORKOUT

Cardio is Hard, Yo

We've got one month to go and now the real work begins. If you enjoyed the quicker-paced super sets or the lung-burning feel of your HIIT workout then stick with that as your main workout. But ALONG with that, we've got to add a little extra push this week. Think of this as the sprinkles on the cupcake. The creamer in your coffee. Your protein in your powder. We have got to up your daily caloric burn again and we have to start right now.

The beauty of this week's work is that you get to be a little creative. The main goal is to increase your caloric burn throughout the day and as long as it meets the main objective (BURN MORE CALORIES), you can do whatever you want.

I've trained bodybuilders that would stand next to their bed and do a ridiculous number of jumping jacks first thing in the morning while their eyes were still closed just so they could get this extra push over with. You could schedule an extra 5-10 minutes on the stair-devil. You could park a block away everywhere you go and get that extra little walk in. Do whatever you want to do just get a little more energy spent.

These small bursts may not seem to be doing much but trust me, they will add up to a bigger energy output at the end of the day – a.k.a. burning more calories. And because it's little

161

by little, you won't even miss them.

Prep Steps for Your Big Day

I know what you're thinking, "Can't someone else do it?" The answer, actually, is yes. If these little spurts don't interest you or perhaps you're just not that creative, why not find someone else to do it?

Look for a boot camp class near you, or get a month pass to a local dance or yoga studio. Pop into some of the classes that your gym offers or do a little YouTubing for some new ways to move. At this point, you've already built up your stabilizer muscles so your risk for injury is greatly reduced and your endurance is such that you can try new things without feeling too silly or weak.

Now is a great time to try a new challenge. It's called cross training and it's one of the best things you can do for your body to avoid hitting a plateau. Just because you attempt a few cross-fit workouts or try some kickboxing classes doesn't mean you have go all in and buy the gear, just find something new and go for it!

Plus, the beauty of attending a class or scheduled workout with an instructor is that you don't have to get creative or over think it. Just follow along and do what they say. In the coming weeks you're going to have plenty of other things to overthink anyway.

Don't worry whether you're on the beat or not, or even if you can't quite keep up, it doesn't matter. The main goal is to increase calorie burn and mistakes burn calories too.

So there you have it – 4 weeks to go and you've got to up the ante and you've got two choices of how you want to do it: look for a million ways to burn a few extra calories or look for a few new challenges that will burn a million calories. Have fun!

4 WEEKS OUT DIET

Taming the Sugar Boogers!

Alright, now that we have a better idea of how much sugar goes into your body, let's talk about what happens when it gets in there.

One thing that is important to remember is that sugar is sugar, whether it's in the little pink bag at the coffee shop or the little blue one. After tracking last week, you may have noticed that it's hiding everywhere disguised as different names like cane sugar, beet sugar, high fructose corn syrup, glucose and fructose to name a few. Whatever name it's called, it all goes through the same route in the body. It's all processed in the liver. With a well-balanced diet, the liver can handle the load of an occasional sugary treat. But when the liver has to work overtime to process the sugar in our juice with breakfast, and then our latte, and then our snack, and then the sugar hidden in our lunch, and then the cookie in the break room, and then our soda with dinner, and then the dessert we "have to have," it just can't keep up.

The overload of sugar begins to infiltrate the bloodstream and nothing good comes of that. Not only do we store more fat but high blood sugar means diabetes and it feeds into several types of cancer.

Because your liver is working so hard to process all of that sugar, it barely has time to process the millions of other toxins

Prep Steps for Your Big Day

we digest or come in contact with so our skin suffers, our energy lulls, the whites of our eyes fade, our hair becomes greasy or dried out, our nails split or break...

...basically, your body ages at an accelerated rate.

So how do we turn back the aging process so you look and feel amazing? It's easy! Sort of.

This week, your goal is to keep your sugar UNDER 50 grams a day. Let me repeat that and this time, read it slow so that it really sinks in.

Under 50 grams.

Of Sugar.

Per day.

This includes any processed, refined, packaged or labeled sugar, NOT any sugar found naturally in fruit or veggies. Bodybuilders and possibly other trainers may be spitting venom at me right now for still allowing that much sugar and fruit in your diet still but I've been in this industry for a very long time and I have helped a lot of people. In my experience, if I tell my clients to go home and clear their cupboards of any and all sugar they only last about 2 days, then it's binge city because your body and brain truly becomes addicted to it. I find it's better to give a budget.

If 50grams doesn't seem like much to you, you're right. By today's standards, it's not, especially when you consider that a can of soda has about 30grams. But here's some news that will make you like me again: you can still have the soda.

Think of your sugar allowance just like your bank account. You've got $50 bucks in there every day, but that $50 (or in this case 50 grams) has got to last you all day – breakfast, lunch, snacks, and dinner. How do you want to spend it?

Do you want to blow 20 grams with the whip cream and caramel drizzle on your coffee? Fine!

Craving a soda with lunch? Go ahead!

But wait! Half way through the day, you remember that there is still some ice cream bars in the freezer for dessert! Have at it! But then you better put the soda back in the fridge at lunch time.

There is not a single thing that is off limits with your 50 grams. Just choose your sugars wisely and stay within your budget and watch what happens. You'll be shocked at the way your skin looks and feels. You'll feel the difference in your hair and nails, and your energy will be high and long-lasting instead of highs and lows. (PS: the lows are usually when we reach for more sugar to pick us back up!)

Remember, don't worry about natural sugars found in fruits and veggies. Remind yourself that you're not depriving yourself of anything, you can have whatever you want. Just like a savvy shopper checks the price tags for the deals, you've got to learn how to make your sugar budget stretch and last all day. Master this (even if it takes you a few weeks) and you'll be ready for what's coming next and looking fierce for your BIG DAY!

4 WEEKS OUT POLISH

Time to Tan

In just one short month you'll be heading down the aisle or to the airport or front and center at your photo shoot, and a little color could be the trick to take your look from pretty to positivity radiant! A month may seem like a long time but to really get a natural-looking, sun-kissed tone (without accidentally over doing it) we need to take some time to build up your tan and avoid blotches, streaks and other mishaps.

No need to call the skin cancer awareness tour bus, I would never suggest you bake yourself in the sun for the next four weeks, artificial or otherwise. The damage will last way past your Big Day and premature wrinkles are the exact opposite of what we're going for here.

Skip the cancer-bulb-in-a-bed and let's experiment with a few different ways to self-tan. If you're rolling your eyes and thinking, "Orange is the new tan?" Relax. Self-tanners have come a long way since their first attempts, no more Umpa-Loompa in a bottle. With a few tips, a little research, and plenty of time to perfect your application technique, you'll be glowing and streak free for your Big Day.

The first step is easy. If you've been a good little reader and following along with your Big Day prep steps so far, you should be consuming a hefty dose of daily anti-oxidants, exfoliating, moisturizing, getting plenty of water and staying

168

away from skin-corrupting fried foods. As important as these things are for your health they are also uber- influential on the tone, texture, and the overall appearance of your skin and the outcome of your tan.

Spray vs. Self-Tan: Spray tans are all the rage these days and they can be a great timesaver over these next few weeks but a spray will require a little prep work before and after. First off, you'll want to be fully exfoliated and hairless before you go, and it can feel a little sticky as it dries, so you'll want to wear loose-fitting clothing.

Most tanning salons have a machine that you stand in (in your birthday suit), push the button, and a barrage of sprayers coat you, but this can leave literal stripes on your skin and it doesn't do well to get into the nooks and crannies of your body. If you're going with a spray tan, do some Yelping for someone who can apply with a hand-held sprayer. The pre-exfoliation step is still crucial for an even tone but a skilled sprayer can make sure it's applied equally and they often use a higher quality formula. Plus, they pay attention not to spray you in the face while you're inhaling, the same cannot be said for a machine!

You'll need to decide where you want your tan lines (if any) so dress appropriately. Don't worry, they've seen it all. Their job is to cover any imperfections and blur out the flaws so be nice and tip well – you don't want to bite the hand that sprays you!

With 4 weeks to go you are going to book two spray tans, the first one you should do now – like tomorrow – so you can watch the results and customize the color. As the treatment sits on your skin, the color gets deeper and deeper so you'll need to decide when to rinse. Showering too soon can make you feel like it did nothing at all and waiting too long before you shower can leave you looking like you've joined the cast of the Jersey Shore.

You'll also be monitoring the fade time for the few days following your spray. To make it last longer, you'll want to lay off the exfoliating for a while. Switch to a moisturizing body wash and just apply gently with your hands, rubbing the skin with your loofa will cause the tan to fade faster and in patches because you'll be schlepping off the inactive skin cells. But, like we already learned, those inactive cells progress at different rates so stay diligent on your moisturizing routine to keep your tan from peeling off like chipped paint. Avoid hot tubs or chemically-treated pools for a while as well until you see how long your skin holds onto the color.

Based on what you learn from your test-drive tan – when to rinse, how long it lasted, which days did it look the best – you'll be better equipped to book your next appointment around your Big Day.

Another option is to peruse the self-tanning aisle at your local beauty or drug store. This is a great option because you have more room to customize and we still have plenty of time to build an even tone. Even if you have a darker complexion there are some on the market that add a little bit of sparkle to your skin as well as softeners and yummy smells so it's an easy step to switch out your regular moisturizer for gradual tanner (gradual tanner, not bronzer – more on that soon).

But don't be duped, more expensive doesn't always mean better because the key is in the application. You could pay top dollar for whatever the latest Kardashian is peddling but still look like you've been finger painted by a three-year-old if not applied correctly.

If you plan to go the self-tan route, invest in an application mitt and take good care of it, you'll be using it every day for the next month. You still want to have a good exfoliating session before you apply. Use your mitt and apply in a circular motion all over your body. You can apply a dab of lotion on the heals/soles of your feet and palms of your hands to keep the color from sticking there and use your tanner lightly

around your knees and elbows as the creases will hold more color and look like ET's skin. Don't forget the backs of your hands and a light sweep over your face and neck, avoiding your eyes.

Now, bronzers are different than tanners. Bronzers do just that, they bronze. Applying a bronzer before you have built up a base tan will make your skin sparkly but that is about it. It doesn't really give a healthy glow it just looks like you went to a Ke$ha party and had a glitter mishap. Think of it as a sparkly nail lacquer, it doesn't look all that pretty on a naked fingernail but with a color under it, it shines.

After a few weeks of building up your tan, then you add a bronze into your routine using your same mitt. Be careful, though, these tend to rub off on clothing and can make your skin look ashy in bright light pictures so use sparingly. Another thing to remember is that the skin on your neck/face will be getting a gradual sun-kissed hue so you'll want to be mindful to change up your foundation or powder makeup to match. You could purchase the next darker shade but after the Big Day it will sit in a drawer. I recommend asking for some darker samples and mix a little bit of the darker pigment with your everyday foundation. It saves a few bucks and gets just the right color!

Prep Steps for Your Big Day

3

3 WEEKS OUT

3 WEEKS OUT WORKOUT

Stay the Course!

Making fitness a part of your everyday life is hard. Being mindful of what you're eating is hard. Trying new things is hard. It's all hard just trying to work it into everyday life, but add to that the fact that your Big Day is just around the corner? That carries its own set of stressors.

These next few weeks your distractions will be multiplied. Your daily endurance will be tested. And your sanity will be tried. But your motivation will not waiver. You know in your heart of hearts that looking (and feeling) your best requires that you make time for you, no matter how many distractions are happening in your world right now.

Slicing out an hour for yourself for a workout could be the only down time you get as your Big Day quickly approaches so don't let that one slide. Do not back burner your goals because other things seem to be more important right now. They are not. Nobody will remember the accent color you chose for the table pieces, or what earrings you wear, but they will remember how radiant and confident you look.

If you haven't already, now is a great time to start using a daily calendar. It takes 5 minutes to download a free scheduler app or a cheap appointment book and it could be the fundamental key to keeping your serenity. Speaking of serenity, how does that prayer go?

Prep Steps for Your Big Day

"Grant me the serenity to accept the things I cannot change, the courage to change the things I can, and the wisdom to know the difference."

Perhaps in this case we can change the wording a bit. As you shuffle your hair appointments, schedule your manicure and trips to the airport we could change it to:

"Give me the time to make it to the appointments I cannot change, the tools to change the appointments I need to, and the wisdom to know the difference." Your workout is one that YOU CANNOT CHANGE.

Block out your workout time on your calendar and if you absolutely must move it, go ahead. But do not delete it! At this point you are surely noticing that you feel better after a workout – less foggy, more energized. So even if that means you have to go to your next appointment marinating in your funk for a while, you'll be in a better mood and far more pro-ductive. Like I always ask my kids and co-workers, "Do you want me smelly and happy, or fresh as a daisy but grumpy because I didn't get my work out?"

Stay the course, dear reader, and just think if you can keep your workout routine on point during this high-stress and busy time, it'll be easy-peasy to keep your routine going when your life slows down a bit!

3 WEEKS OUT DIET

Just a Little Nip/Tuck

So, last week you got your sugar intake limited to only 50 grams a day. Nothing was off limits. You had a balance of 50 in your sugar bank account, a daily budget, and you were thoughtful on where you wanted to spend it. Maybe it was challenging for you. Maybe not. But hopefully, being thoughtful of labels and sugar intake is something that will stick with you for the rest of your days. But now, back to the task at hand – making sure you look your absolute best in just 3 short weeks!

If you've mastered the 50g of sugar task then this week won't be so bad. This week, we just need to do a little nip/tuck to that sugar budget of yours. Instead of 50 grams a day and unlimited fruits, we're making a little cutback. This week, skim your intake to only 30 grams of sugar per day and the only thing that is strictly off limits is alcohol. This may be easier for some than others, but if you need more help in kicking that habit, I'm afraid that is out of my jurisdiction. If the struggle to stay away from alcohol (any and all) for the next few weeks is too big to manage than I encourage you to seek professional help. I've had clients who were ready and willing to do anything to prepare for their Big Day, they cleaned up their diet, they were diligent with their workouts, they got good nutrition all day long, and chose to save their sugar budget for a few drinks at night and followed my plan to a T, except when it came time to cut the alcohol. Because when the shakes and restlessness set in, it was a scary realization how much dependency had developed.

Detoxing aside, it's a small adjustment to the changes you've already made and it will have a huge impact on your skin, energy and waistline over the next few weeks.

If cutting back to only 30 grams of sugar is dramatic from what you were used to consuming, you may not feel like your best self so brace yourself for a little bit of crabbiness or bloating the first day or so as the yeast in your gut levels out. You see, yeast in the body is a good thing, but it feeds on any and all kinds of sugar, and if you're used to feeding it too much, your body's balance will be sent all out of whack. Bringing it back into whack can be little uncomfortable at first, but it gets better, I promise!

You may have some bloating around your middle and lower abdomen that you didn't even know was there – after just a few weeks of reduced sugar, you'll be shocked at the definition in your mid-section. Just don't give into sugar cravings! Your gut may tell your brain that you NEED it, but don't listen, that is just the starving yeast talking. Reach for a piece of fruit to keep the cravings at bay.

Remember, the only thing off limits is alcohol and your sugar bank account just shrunk a little from 50 grams a day to 30 grams a day. No biggie. Good luck!

3 WEEKS OUT POLISH

Smile Time!

You know what goes great with stained, yellow teeth? Nothing! Yes it's time we shine up your pearly whites for your Big Day and starting now, 3 weeks away from the Big Day, will give you plenty of time to make them sparkle and give any irritation of the gums (a common side effect to whitening treatments) time to recuperate. Don't worry, it's not going to hurt but sensitive gums and teeth may become a little touchy so by starting now, you'll be able to have plenty of downtime between short treatments and still get the same effect as one long, powerful treatment that a professional offers and for a fraction of the cost.

So what's the difference? Not much. Most over the counter whitening products, like tooth strips or trays, use a solution that is about 3.5-10% hydrogen peroxide to bleach the tooth. It's the same active ingredient in the solutions you'd get if you had it done professionally but the concentration is much higher, ranging from 25-40%.

Starting now with an inexpensive treatment at a lower concentration will help keep sensitive teeth happy because it's not nearly as aggressive and any pain usually goes away when the product is removed. You can rinse the treatment, let the soft tissue or grumpy tooth recover, and then do it again in a day or two without doing any permanent harm to the teeth or

Prep Steps for Your Big Day

gums. Plus, all those healthy foods and antioxidants you're ingesting now will speed up your recovery time!

You'll want to do a little research before you go to the drug store but since the active ingredient is the same in all home products, it's going to come down to what you feel like doing – drooling with a tray in your mouth or peeling a slimy sticker off your teeth. Neither process is very attractive and costs range from $10 to $30. But it's a one-time investment so I say splurge a little bit here. The higher end ones tend to have a better consistency!

So here we go! Three weeks until your Big Day. Say cheese!

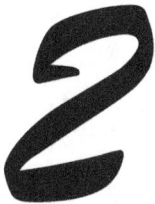

2 WEEKS OUT

2 WEEKS OUT WORKOUT

In and Out

It's almost here! Finding time and energy for your workouts is probably getting a little tricky as we head into crunch time so for this next to last week, shift your focus to in and out. No, not the burger joint, in and out as in – get your work- out in and get out.

This week we need to use moves that will give us the most bang for our buck. We won't get hung up on sets, reps, class times, waiting for equipment, etc. Just get in and get out!

If you can still make it to your regular workout routine then carry on! But carving out time to drive to the gym or to your favorite class can get tough these last few weeks and skipping your workout completely is not an option. Do these quick routines or something similar in the corner of your garage or living room. Whenever and wherever you can find a few minutes to fit it in, do it! These Till Failure Workouts will only take you about 15-20 minutes and require nothing but your body and space. Try it once in the morning and again later in the day if you can to keep your caloric burn ignited.

The idea here is TO WORK TILL FAILURE, not till tired.

Working till failure means you should be thinking: "I cannot do this move one more single time!"

Prep Steps for Your Big Day

Working till failure means not counting.

Working till failure means not using a timer.

Working till failure means listening to your body.

Working till failure means the muscle is absolutely fatigued and cannot continue.

Think you get it? It's hard not to count and it's hard not to work in the parameters of a timed set. And every body is different. Your till failure is different than my till failure and on some moves, to get to your till failure, you might spend your entire workout time on just one of these combo moves, and that's okay.

Pick a few from these lists and have at it! Remember, no timers and no counting. You're just working, working, working until you can't work no more!

Combo Moves to Failure:

Do each move as many as times as you possibly can. If you poop out on just one part of the exercise, then that means you're done!

Combo Move 1) 3 pushups (on knees or toes), followed by 3 knee tucks – like the bottom part of a burpee. Hands stay still, knees come to chest and push back out to a plank position.

Combo Move 2) 5 full-range bodyweight squats, followed by 5 jump squats.

Combo Move 3) 8 pulses in a side plank, rotate sides (without dropping), 8 pulses on other side.

Combo Move 4) Stationary lunge for 3 pulses, bring back leg forward for a front kick. Fatigue each side.

Combo Move 5) Push-up (knees or toes) followed by down-dog push-up (on toes). Tuck chin, lift tailbone to sky and perform a push up as if you're trying to touch the crown of your head to the floor.

Combo Move 6) Perform a wide-stance squat, rise up and add a side kick left. Repeat with side kick right.

Combo Move 7) Perform 3 body-weight squats followed by one explosive start jump (spread your arms and legs like a star fish in the air).

Combo Move 8) Ice skaters for 4 counts (that means right, left, right, left) followed by 4 tuck jumps (knees come to chest).

Single Body Weight Moves to Failure:

Pushups

Wide stance squats with both heels off the ground

Plank

Military style sit ups

Wall squats

Remember, everything you do, you do until muscle failure whether that means 5 repetitions or 50. Just get in and get out. You've only got 2 weeks until your Big Day!

2 WEEKS OUT DIET

So Long Sweet Tooth

O kay, we cut your sugar intake from whatever you were consuming before to 50 grams a day and nothing was off limits. Then, we whittled it down to 30 grams of sugar a day with alcohol being your only deal breaker. This week, with only 2 weeks until your Big Day, we bring out the big guns. NO MORE SUGAR.

Go ahead take a moment to let that sink in. This week and next there will be no sugar in your diet unless it comes in the form of fruit. That's it. That's all.

Time to rethink your coffee order.

If you've been paying attention, you've already cut out breads for the interim. No alcohol right now. You're not eating fried foods anymore, and your dinner plate is a colorful blend of veggies and lean proteins. Friend, you're already practically paleo so this week will be easy-peasy and it is the final push on your preparations to looking your absolute best on your Big Day!

Cut the sugar. Eat more fruit. No need to keep repeating my- self. If you want to look your best, this is what you've got to do. I can feel you cursing at me under your breath but I know you'll do fine. You've already come this far, a few weeks without sugar isn't going to kill you. Although I'm feeling as though you may be harboring thoughts of killing me?

2 WEEKS OUT POLISH

Sweet Dreams

T wo weeks to go and stress is your middle name. But stress can wreak havoc on your skin, your energy, and your sleep. It'll be hard to walk down the aisle carrying those heavy bags under your eyes so let's take some time this week to focus on sleep and stress reduction so you can get some good Z's.

Of course it's important for your health but just take moment to visualize how you might look after 2 weeks of stressed-out sleep deprivation. This is in the polish section for a reason.

No matter what your Big Day is, you're obviously crazy excited about it or else you wouldn't have put this much preparation time into it, so as it gets closer your probably getting more and more excited/nervous so I've got a few tips to help you calm your mind, find some peace, and focus during these next 2 crazy weeks.

First of all, don't discount a good yoga class. You don't have to be a yogi to reap the benefits of not looking at your phone for an hour. If relaxation is what you're looking for, seek out a class or YouTube video with titles like "Beginner," "Restorative," or "Gentle." These imply that the moves will be done slowly with a focus on meditation of the mind not power of the body. Heading to a power yoga or hot yoga is great if you're already into the practice of yoga but expect a sweaty workout, not a restful, quieting practice.

Next, and probably a bit easier to incorporate at this point, is just introducing some breathing practices to quiet your mind and calm your body before bed. Here are few of my favorites:

Lying flat on your back or with a pillow under your head/ neck, place your hand on your belly button. As you inhale deeply, imagine sending all of the air right to your belly button. Your hand should rise and fall with your breath. Repeat 3-5 times.

Next, move your hand a few inches up until it rests on your bottom rib. Send all of the air there, again feeling the hand rise and fall. Repeat 3-5 times.

Then, move your hand up to the center of your chest, right where a necklace would lay, your décolletage or center between your collar bones. Send all of the air there. Repeat 3-5 times.

Lastly, try taking a small sip of air to the belly button, a small sip of air to the ribs, and a small sip of air to the chest, then exhale completely. Repeat 3-5 times.

I almost always end my yoga classes with this technique. Maybe that's why no one ever wants to get up after class.

Or try this simple trick:

Lying in any position you feel comfortable, breathe in through the nose for 4 counts and out through the mouth for 4 counts. You can experiment with counting to 5 or 6, maybe even 8, as you start to calm down. But anytime you feel your mind start to wander, bring it back to your counting.

That's it. That's all. Ever wonder why counting sheep got so much credit? This is it. Taken right from the therapist couch, a simple counting distraction can calm the nervous system and help to release sleep inducing chemicals in the brain.

And one more option, try inhaling as much as you can, and when you think you've reached your max, try to get one more sip of air in. Then exhale as much as you can, and when you think you've reached your max, try getting one more sip of air out. Try this for a few minutes before bed to clear your mind and reset your stress levels.

If these aren't doing the trick, a trip to your local health food store for some calming teas or a small dose of melatonin might help. I don't recommend any over the counter sleep aids because they all have the same active ingredient, diphen-hydramine, and it takes FOREVER for that shiz to leave your body, sometimes up to 3 days! Good sleep is vital to getting all your stuff done but dragging around like a zombie for 3 days is the exact opposite. So try other methods before you reach for anything PM.

Other pharmaceuticals or treatments are out of my jurisdiction so talk to your doctor or naturopath if you're really having a hard time getting good Z's because it really is so important in your overall health, your fitness journey, and your Big Day look.

Prep Steps for Your Big Day

1

1 WEEK OUT

1 WEEK OUT WORKOUT

Give Grace

With 1 week to go until your Big Day, you've probably got plenty to do – last minute packing, planning, and primping – and if you're following along with the diet portion of the 1 Week Out section, you're going to need to conserve your energy.

A short walk to clear your head or a gentle yoga practice would be okay but as for an all-out sweat session, give yourself some grace this week and focus on your other chores. If you do find time to hit the gym, go light and easy, maybe just cruise on the stationary bike to keep the muscles loose.

Not only is this to maintain your sanity but really, to look and feel your best next week, a little rest can go a long way. Don't worry, the changes you've seen in your body won't go away in just one week.

Just don't forget to get back on the workout wagon after your Big Day passes!

1 WEEK OUT DIET

Drying Out

Y ou have one week left and today you need to ask yourself
a very important question:

Do you really want to go through with this?

You could change your mind right now and nobody would get hurt. Everything will be fine and you'll just pick up and carry on as normal. I'm talking, of course, about cutting water weight. There is a stealthy little trick in the fitness and beauty world that can lean you out, create more muscle definition, and even drop a few pounds quickly. But it can be dangerous. And this is NOT a way to lose weight for the long term. This is NOT part of a healthy lifestyle and I do NOT recommend doing this cut unless you are truly aware of the risks and are in good health.

Do you ever notice that your tummy is a little flatter in the morning, or that your shoulders and arms have better defini- tion? You may not have ever connected that it usually comes after an evening of dining on salty foods or alcohol, which depletes the subcutaneous layer of water, thus tightening the skin and showing more of the muscle you've worked so hard to achieve. Or have you ever weighed yourself in the morning and seen a substantial loss from the night before? Don't break into your happy dance, this isn't real fat loss. It's water! And it can shift up to 10 pounds, depending on your intake and retention.

Prep Steps for Your Big Day

Water weight is a tricky thing and manipulating it requires lots of knowledge of your own body. Wrestlers and fighters cut water before a match to land in the weight class they want to be in and then quickly rehydrate so they can perform at high athletic levels. Fitness and figure competitors cut for the day of show to get the most definition possible. And if you decide to cut water for your Big Day, you will see tighter definition and smaller waist line.

With that said, if you are going to do it, there is a right way and a lot of wrong ways to dry out. Follow this plan for the safest way to cut and I repeat, this is NOT a way to live. And heed my disclaimer – this can be dangerous.

If you've followed along and cut out the nasty oils, drastically reduced your sugar, revved up your intake of fruits and veggies and put a hold on the breads for a while, you should be seeing some pretty impressive things from your body. As long as you're getting plenty of nutrients from your foods and you are in good health you should be able to do this with no problems. But remember, cut at your own risk.

Cutting water weight can put a strain on your kidney and liver function, and any achy joint you have will be amplified due to the buildup of toxins that aren't being flushed out. Be prepared to feel a little creaky (and cranky) as the week goes on. Also, you'll see that in this last week's workout section, doesn't have any workouts. That's because your body will not be able to perform the way it is used to, so don't even try. You'll be tired, sluggish and you may experience some headaches. So now that you know all the awful things that come along with dehydrating and you still want to go through with it, here's how to do it somewhat safely:

We start by working backwards from your Big Day and flood the body with a ridiculous amount of water, then we cut each day's intake by half. So if your event is on a Saturday we start the Sunday before by consuming about 2 gallons of water. It's a lot. And you'll spend most of the day looking for the closest restroom. But it is absolutely the most crucial step! We want to flood the kidneys to such a level that they will be able to sustain a drought without causing any damage. The rest of the week is pointless if you can't execute this step, and you run a much higher risk of danger to the kidneys. So you must start with 2 gallons of water (more if you can) about 6 days out and cut your intake by half each day. So your week would look like this:

Sunday – 2 gallons

Monday – 1 gallon

Tuesday   –   ½

gallon

Wednesday – ¼ gallon or 4 8oz. cups

Thursday – 16oz or 2 cups of water. That's it. All day. Make it last.

Friday – sips or ice chips to wet your whistle, but that's it!

Saturday – It's Your Big Day! Start with 8-16oz in the morning to revitalize your skin and energy and continue with cupful's throughout the day.

By Saturday morning you'll be tired, achy, cranky and head-achy so quickly begin to rehydrate. Even if your event is later in the day, you can start drinking again because the fluids will go the places that need it the most first – your kidneys and internal organs – and you won't see that in a wedding gown. You'll still maintain a flattering stomach and muscle definition for most of the day until you are fully hydrated. But be care-ful, as the day goes on things will be hectic so don't forget to get your water in. The last thing you want is to pass out or be rushed to an IV on your Big Day so don't forget to rehydrate!

1 WEEK OUT POLISH

All the Finishing Touches

It's almost time! You have worked so hard and done so many wonderful things for your body, hair, and skin that you must be loving what you see in the mirror right now! In just a few short days it will be your time in the spotlight! Whatever your Big Day is, you will walk with confidence. Now it's time to put together all of those finishing touches that will make you shine and this week. Timing is everything!

If you decide to have your nails done by a professional it's okay to book your mani-pedi appointment early in the week as they are sure to last through your Big Day and if you have any chips or breaks, they'll have plenty of time to fix it. If full-on fake nails aren't your thing at least go for gel polish as it lasts much longer than regular nail lacquer and doesn't chip off. It will cost a bit more, but worth every penny to not have to keep retouching throughout the week.

If you're more of a DIYer you'll want to wait until later in the week to apply your coats at home so they don't chip. Gel polish is available now at drugstores, and again, paying a bit extra for the gel polish to prevent chips is totally worth it. Don't worry about staying in the lines if you're no Picasso, if polish gets on your surrounding skin, simply wipe off with a Q-tip dipped in polish remover or wait for it to dry completely and give it a little extra scrub in the shower.

Prep Steps for Your Big Day

If you're opting for a spray tan you'll need to time it just right based on what you learned during your trial tan. You'll have to be exfoliated and hairless before you go so book any waxing or sugaring appointments first. If you're shaving, you'll want to wait to spray until closer to the Big Day or you'll need to deal with grow out and you'll just shave your tan right off.

Schedule your spray tan the day before your Big Day and get a good shave just before you go in so you don't have any 5 o'clock shadow. Remember, the longer it sits on your skin the deeper the color, so when you like what you see, and hop in the shower for a rinse to deactivate the tanner.

If you've been building up your base with your own self-tanner, now is the time to incorporate a bronzer. Just be careful as they tend to rub off on fabrics. One trick that might help is to apply your bronzer and then wear a bathrobe or an old towel around for a while, that way any of the sparkle that is going to rub off, will rub off on that fabric and not your pretty (and possibly expensive) outfit.

As for your hair and makeup, maybe you hire a pro to manage that department or maybe you've got your look dialed in. Whatever you decide, the prep work you've done thus far by cutting out the oils, increasing your water, and nutrients – Including those awesome anti-oxidants – pretty much guarantees your skin will look amazing and your hair is healthy and strong.

It's Your Big Day!

You did it! During a crazy, busy time when you had a million other things to worry about, you got it done. If you can make these healthy habits a part of your life in the middle of a storm, you'll have no trouble at all keeping your focus during calmer waters.

Enjoy your wonderful day, whatever it might be! Walk with confidence and grace and be proud.

You may not be exactly where you want to be with only 10 weeks under your belt but you've come a long way and what you see in the mirror is the direct result of your hard work and dedication. Just imagine the results if you stayed on this track for a little while longer!

After today, you can go back to eating whatever the heck you want, quit worrying about your exfoliation routine, and stop eating all those pesky antioxidant- rich foods – but I'll warn you, it won't be pretty. You'll notice your eyes aren't quiet as bright, your skin will dull and you'll feel sluggish and lazy.

My advice is: scan the calendar for your next Big Day. Maybe a friend's wedding or an upcoming trip or maybe a holiday party you want to look great for and go back to the beginning of this book and begin your Big Day prep again!

Or the opposite might happen. You'll notice that you look and feel the best you have ever felt and continue integrating all of the steps you've learned so far into your everyday life, maybe with a few cheats here and there and that's okay. It's a lot harder to stay motivated without an impending Big Day coming at you.

And now, my dearly beloved reader, as we gather here today to finish this book…

Just kidding.

But in all seriousness, thank you for letting me be a small part of your Big Day. I hope you like what you see in the mirror and that you've grown in your fitness and wellness journey. Be proud. Walk with confidence. You are beautiful.

If you are so inclined to share your photos or stories of your journey with me, it would be an honor! Email me at kim@ kimatthegym.com, tag #kimatthegym on Instagram, or find me on Facebook at Kim Rose/Kimatthegym

Have a wonderful Big Day!

SUCCESS STORIES

Prep Steps for Your Big Day

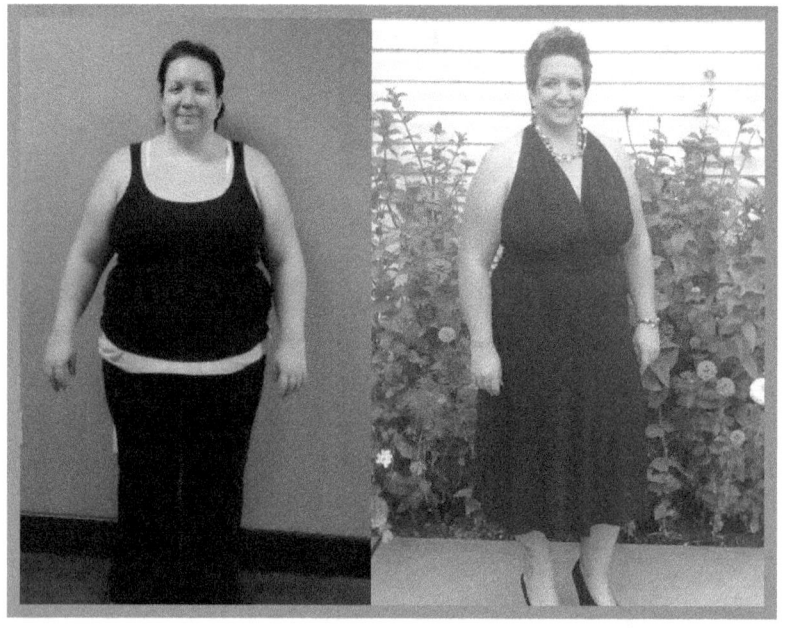

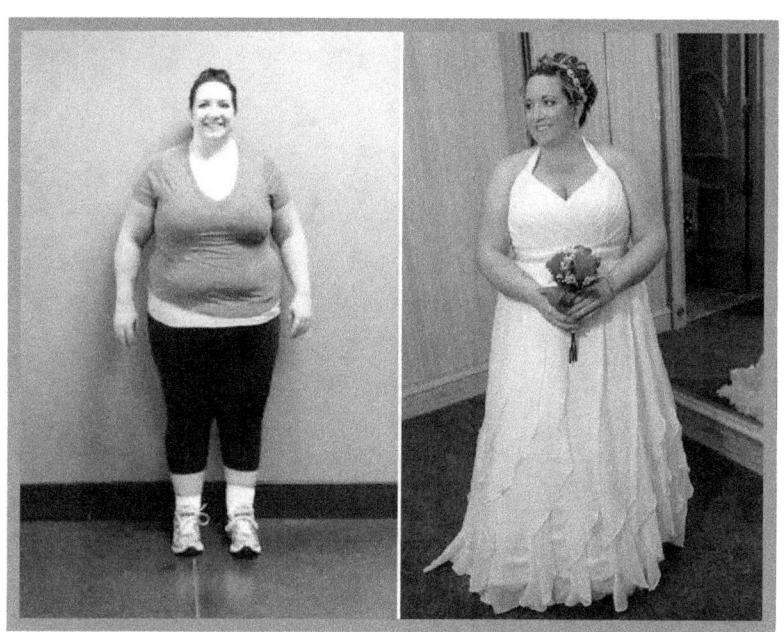

BRANDI

Brandi first came to me when she knew she was going to be a bridesmaid in her brother's wedding. After working together for 12 weeks, she fit comfortably into that little black dress and looked stunning.

A few years later, after taking time off due to serious and scary health issues, Brandi met the love of her life. She called me again and we got to work to prep for her own wedding day. She says, "It was harder this time but I had to stay focused and push through because it was important for me to feel beautiful about myself inside and out."

ELVIRA

"My Big Day was a local fashion show, a fundraiser for Youth Diabetes Programs in our area. I'm not sure how I got roped into it and I was so nervous. But by the time of the show I felt so beautiful and I walked the runway with so much confidence. I really loved myself and it showed."

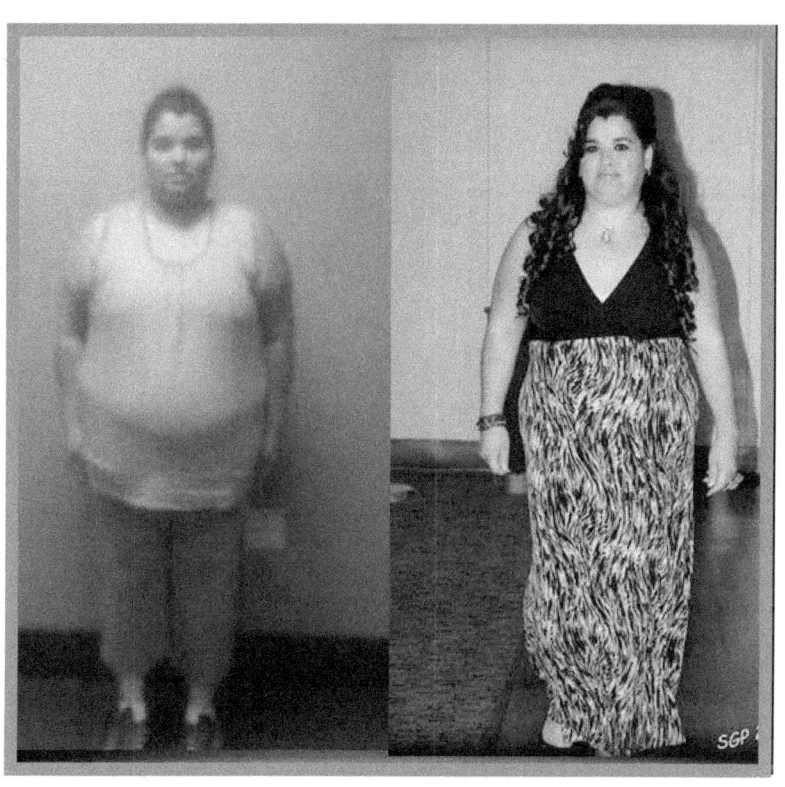

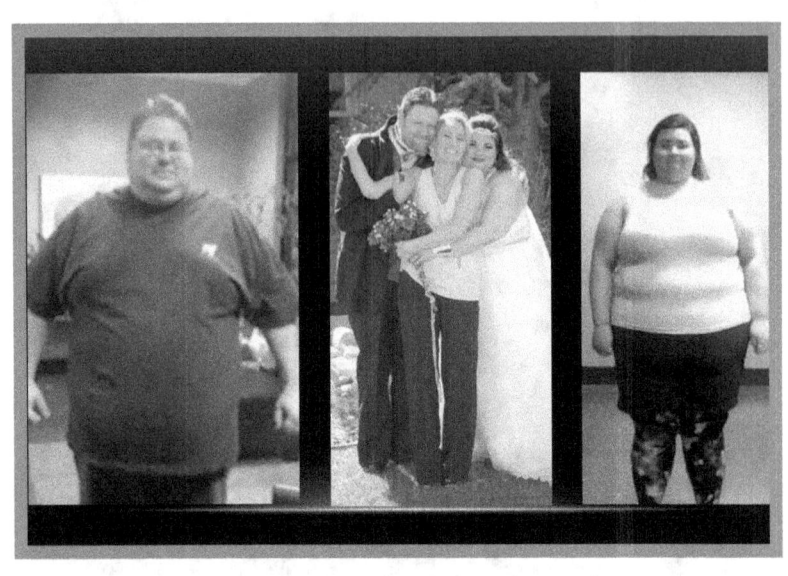

MICHAEL AND KELLY

I will never forget the day I met Michael. He was 420lbs and didn't make eye contact with me, his eyes were fixed on the floor as I asked pointed questions about what made him decide it's time for a change. We had been together almost every day for about a year both in private and in group classes when Kelly joined the studio.

She too was quiet and reserved and made the corner in the back of the room her own. I didn't think much of it when the two of them had started hanging around after class, Michael had already come so far on his journey and he was so good at supporting others. The staring contest with the floor had been long over with his new confidence.

A few months later, several of us were participating in a community 5k when I saw Michael and Kelly holding hands as they crossed the finish line. I thought my heart was going to explode! These two beautiful people had found each other through health and grew their friendship through encouragement and patience and kindness.

A few years later, both still pursuing new challenges, Kelly has completed several 10k runs and Michael became a group fitness instructor, they asked me to marry them. I almost declined out of fear that I would cry too much while performing the vows and ruin their Big Day and I did cry. A lot. But it didn't ruin anything. It was a beautiful day and the highest compliment I have ever received.

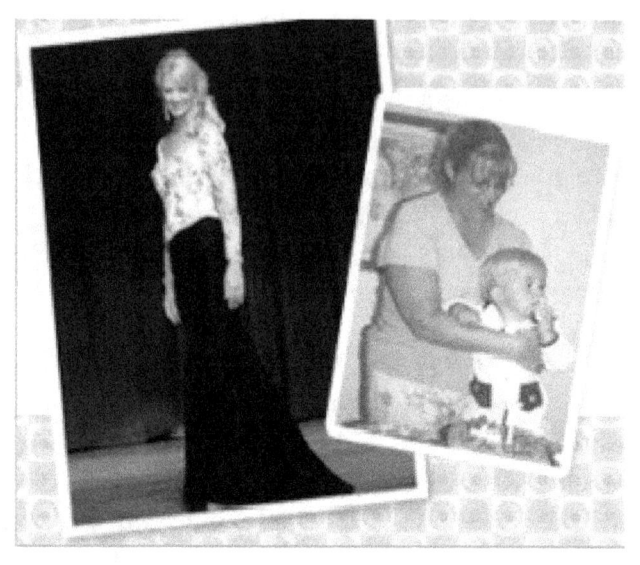

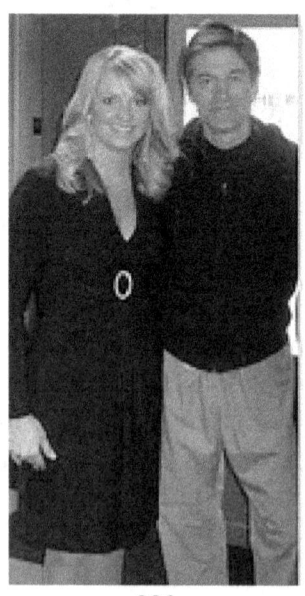

JILL KNAPP

After losing 100 pounds, it was a true honor when my dear friend and client asked me to help her prepare for the stage in the Mrs. America Pageant. What makes Jill's story so unique is that she had been diagnosed with Type 2 Diabetes and through healthy changes, new exercise habits and a true understanding of her body, she was able to get off of her insulin completely!

With her astounding success story and her beauty inside and out, it came as no surprise when Dr. Oz asked her to be on his show. So...we had another Big Day to prep for!

Jill has gone onto be an advocate for diabetes education and travels the country motivating others. See her page at www.GetUpandGetMoving.net

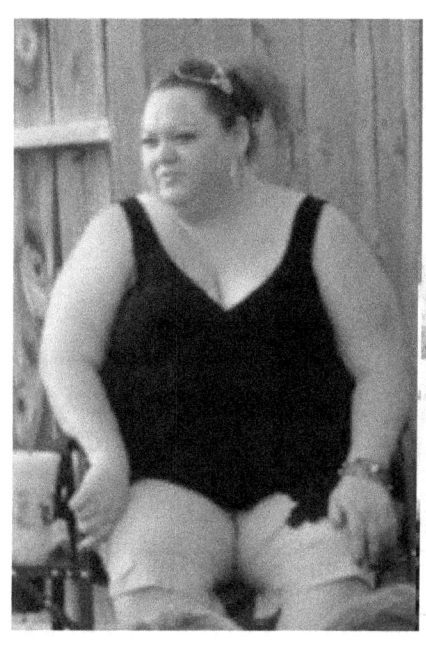 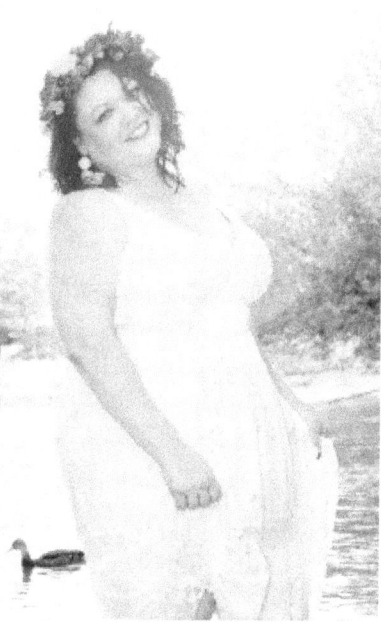

TINA CLARKE

When meeting new clients, I always ask them what they are preparing for. More often than not, there is a Big Day looming that they want to get ready for. But I will never forget the day I met Tina.

I asked- "So is there something coming up that you want to get ready for?"

She said "No?" Kind of confused.

And I replied "Ahhh...LIFE! You want to get ready for LIFE!

I didn't know it at the time but those words resonated with her as she shares that story often. Together we navigated through some pretty heavy issues from a family history of obesity to food addiction (that she now openly shares with others who struggle), to finding new ways to move a back and body that, somedays, didn't want to move.

And then one day, when her confidence was at an all-time high, she booked a session with professional photographer for no particular reason...except to capture that beautiful, glowing smile.

She made her own Big Day to prep for!